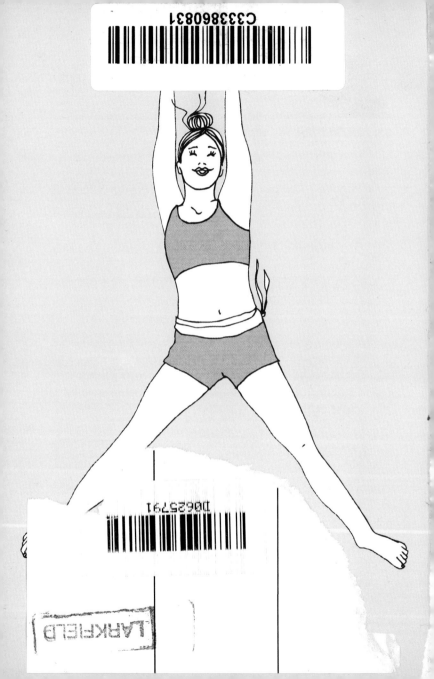

THIS IS A CARLTON BOOK

This edition published in 2016 by Carlton Books
an imprint of the Carlton Books Group
20 Mortimer Street
London W1T 3JW

First edition published in 2004
Second edition published in 2011

Text copyright © Carlton Books Group 2004
Design copyright © Carlton Books Group 2016

A CIP catalogue record for this book is available from the British Library.

ISBN 978 1 78097 703 4

Printed and bound in China

Illustrations: Sam Loman

This book reports information and opinions which may be of general interest to the
reader. It is advisory only and is not intended to serve as a medical textbook or other
procedural guide, or as a substitute for consultation with a physician in relation to
any symptoms that may require diagnosis and medical attention. The information and
opinions contained herein are those solely of the author and not those of the publishers
who disclaim any responsibility for any consequences that may result from any use of or
reliance thereon by the reader.

HEALTH
HACKS

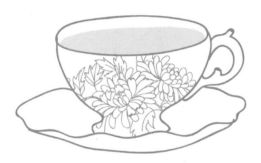

500
SIMPLE SOLUTIONS
THAT PROVIDE BIG BENEFITS

Esme Floyd

CARLTON
BOOKS

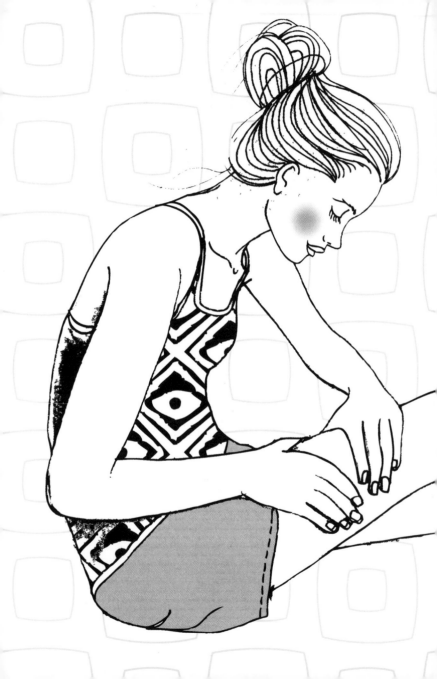

CONTENTS

INTRODUCTION

Did you know that wrapping presents could help you burn 100 calories an hour, or that butter could actually be better for you than low-fat alternatives?

Here we've gathered together 500 health hacks to help you stay happy and healthy in every area of your life. Simply read through the book or dip in and out according to how you feel. From hayfever cures to workout wisdom, from travel problems to beating stress, the book contains advice to help make your life brighter and better.

TOP TEN HEALTH HACKS

GO NUTTY FOR WEIGHT LOSS
(see Calories, page 9)

BUILD 24-CARROT BONES
(see Miracle foods, page 19)

HAVE A BRAZILIAN
(see Energy-boosters, page 29)

DON'T LET SHOULDERS CREEP UP ON YOU
(see Posture, page 34)

HOLD YOUR TONGUE
(see Sleep, page 42)

DROP A SIZE TO BE KNEE-WISE
(see Arthritis, page 52)

ROOT OUT SICKNESS
(see Nausea, page 66)

USE SUNFLOWERS TO SHRINK FAT
(see Cellulite, page 88)

GET A-GRADE SKIN
(see Skin health, page 101)

TREAT TRAVEL SICKNESS WITH GINGER
(see Travel, page 126)

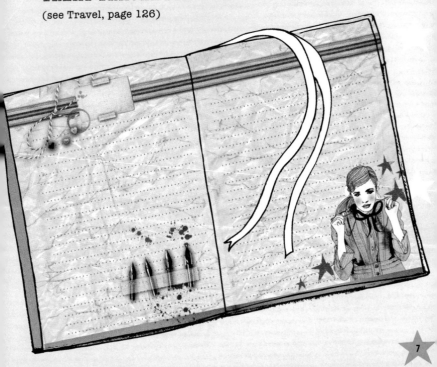

DIET & NUTRITION

ALCOHOL

AVOID FLUSHING AWAY FOLATE

Alcohol reduces folic acid and vitamin B6, both of which are essential for the body to protect against a range of diseases and conditions, including breast cancer. If you drink regularly, make sure you're getting enough folic acid (found in liver, fortified breakfast cereals, leafy green vegetables and numerous supplements).

DRINK YOURSELF PINK

Drinking just one or two glasses of wine a day could cut your risk of heart disease by up to a third, and red and rosé wines may be even more beneficial than white wine because of the higher levels of antioxidants they contain.

CALORIES

GO THE EXTRA MILE

Experts suggest that to lose weight you need to eliminate 500 calories a day. For most people, this means an hour of walking at a rate of 12 minutes per mile.

CHEW THOSE CALORIES AWAY

Replacing a packet of full-sugar chewing gum with a sugar-free variety could save 100 calories.

GET FULL WITH THE FIZZ

Swapping a sugary drink or glass of wine for sparkling water at lunchtime could save hundreds of calories over the week.

GO NUTTY FOR WEIGHT LOSS

Nuts might be high in calories, but thanks to the construction of their cell walls, our body can't access them all, which means they're even healthier than once thought. Almonds are particularly nutritious.

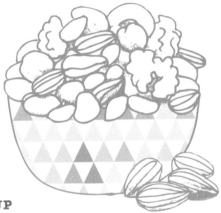

CLEAN UP TO BURN UP

Cleaning and general housework around the home, such as mopping the floor or vacuuming the carpet, burns off an incredible 233 calories an hour, which is the equivalent of a bagel.

GO SKINNY TO SKIM OFF CALORIES

Choosing a coffee with skimmed milk rather than whole milk could save you the same amount of calories as 20 minutes of moderate cycling.

SHAVE PORTIONS TO SHED INCHES

A great way to shave off calories without losing the taste of your food is to eat smaller portions. Reducing the size of a steak from 150g to 75g (5oz to 3oz) could save more than 200 calories.

FAVOUR LOW-FAT FILLINGS
Changing the mayonnaise in your sandwich from full fat to low fat could save the same amount of calories as you'd burn up doing an extra hour at work.

WRAP IT UP
Did you know you can use up 100 calories an hour wrapping presents? What a perfect excuse to buy gifts!

THINK THIN AND TALL
People perceive tall, thin glasses to hold more than short ones, and drink 20% more from stubbier ones. For high-calorie drinks, like fruit juice, smoothies or alcohol, use tall, narrow glasses. You'll think you drank more than you actually did.

TAKE YOUR TIME IN THE BATHROOM
Don't skimp on getting glam before you go out. Doing your hair and make-up helps you burn off a fantastic 166 calories an hour.

CHOLESTEROL

GET IN PEAK FORM WITH PECANS
Adding pecans to your diet not only lowers total cholesterol and levels of LDL, or 'bad' cholesterol, but can also help maintain HDL, or 'good' cholesterol, in the blood.

SHARE THE CHARDONNAY
It might sound an unlikely ally in the fight against cholesterol, but research has revealed that just a glass of Chardonnay a day might help your body get rid of damaging cholesterol.

HAVE A MINI-DRIVE

More frequent mini-meals or light snacks that spread out your calorie intake evenly throughout the entire day help maintain a steady balance in blood chemistry, avoiding peaks and dips in blood sugar and lowering cholesterol.

PRUNE BACK BLOOD CHOLESTEROL

Prunes contain high levels of antioxidants that help lower stored levels of damaging LDL, making them a perfect quick snack.

BOTTOMS UP FOR BETTER BALANCE

One or two glasses of antioxidant-rich wine or beer a day will not only encourage your body to produce HDL – the antho-cyanins and other antioxidants they contain can also lower LDL.

SWEAT HEALTH TROUBLES AWAY

Physical exercise is a factor in reducing the levels of destructive LDL in the bloodstream, thus restoring a good cholesterol balance and helping your system maintain health. For the best results, aim for between three and four workouts every week.

GIVE YOUR LIVER A BREAK

Only about 20% of the cholesterol in the body is ingested directly through the diet. A whopping 80% is produced by the liver in response to processed foods and saturated fats. Eating fruits, vegetables, wholegrains and oily fish stops your liver having to work so hard.

JUICE AWAY BAD CHOLESTEROL

Drinking three small glasses of orange juice every day could not only reduce LDL levels in the blood but also boost levels of HDL by up to a fifth, making it a great choice for heart health.

DEHYDRATION

DRINK UP TO TONE UP

Drinking the right amount of water helps maintain muscle tone by giving muscles their natural ability to contract, so making sure you don't get dehydrated helps you tone up and strengthen up, too.

DON'T WAIT TILL YOU'RE THIRSTY

If you feel thirsty, you're already dehydrated. Aim to drink little and often throughout the day so you never get to the stage where you feel thirsty.

COUNT TO EIGHT

Water suppresses the appetite naturally and helps the body metabolize stored fat, actually reducing fat deposits. Make sure you get your eight glasses a day if you want to stay slim.

GULP DOWN A CLEAR WINNER

Alcohol and drinks that contain caffeine, especially coffee and colas, cause rather than protect against dehydration. Choose plain water instead.

GO RAW FOR GOOD FLUID RESERVES

You can supplement your fluid intake by eating raw fruits and vegetables, such as tomatoes, broccoli, lettuce, carrots, watermelon, grapefruit and apples. All of these fruits and vegetables contain high levels of water.

STAY SHARP WITH REGULAR SIPPING

A major effect of dehydration is on concentration. If you're dehydrated, you'll stop being able to think clearly and experts believe this is why many people have an afternoon lull. To keep alert, drink water throughout the day.

PROTECT MUSCLES WITH WATER

Water in the body binds to muscle glycogen at a rate of 4 grams to every gram of glycogen. If you starve your body of water or food, these groups are split up and although you might lose weight, it's not the right weight to lose.

DON'T WATER DOWN YOUR HEALTH

Water makes up between 50% and 70% of the human body and is the essential constituent of blood, lymph, digestive juices, urine and perspiration. Without it, your body simply can't function, and experts recommend you drink 1.5-2 litres (2½-3½ pints) spread throughout the day.

DAMP DOWN ON DEHYDRATION

When exercising in hot or humid conditions, you can lose 2-3 litres (3½-5¼ pints) of water per hour, leaving an average-sized woman dehydrated after only half an hour's activity. Drinking two glasses of water before you work out sets you up for a successful session.

CLEAR UP YOUR MEMORY

It might not sound much, but a mere 2% drop in your body's water levels – 1 litre (1¾ pints) of water for someone who weighs 68kg (10st 10lb/150lbs) – results in short-term memory impairment, trouble with basic maths and difficulty in focusing.

SHIFT MORE WEIGHT BY DRINKING UP

Dehydration can slow down metabolism as it springs the body into starvation mode and holds onto fat cells that contain high levels of fluids. So drink up to keep your metabolism rate high.

DETOX

GET ENERGETIC WITH A CLEANSING TONIC

Try this cleansing tonic to help strengthen your liver: 200ml (7fl oz) spring water, juice of a lemon, pinch of powdered ginger, 1 table-spoon flaxseeds, 1 teaspoon psyllium powder.

PRACTISE YOUR BRUSHSTROKE

Dry body brushing before showering has been shown to stimulate lymphatic flow and circulation and remove dead skin cells. You'll need a soft bristle brush with a long detachable handle, to enable you to reach right down your back.

DRESS IN LEMON AND GINGER

Avoid caffeine, alcohol, refined sugar and salt. Instead, season your food with lemon juice, garlic, ginger or cayenne pepper, all of which support the detox process while adding flavour.

PURIFY WITH A HOME BREW

Make a purifying herb tea from 1 teaspoon each of nettle, peppermint, dandelion root and red clover combined in a saucepan with 3 cups of cold water. Bring to the boil, reduce the heat and simmer for 15 minutes. Strain and sweeten with apple juice if required.

SPLASH OUT WITH SALSA

Use hot tomato salsa as an alternative to butter or mayonnaise to add spicy flavour to your baked potatoes and as a piquant accompaniment to meat and fish. It tastes delicious and the chilli and tomatoes help your body detox.

FL-OAT TOXINS AWAY

Oats are a great food for detoxing as they help the body flush out toxins as well as releasing their energy slowly into the body to prevent cravings (unrolled oats are more effective at this) and lowering cholesterol in the blood.

FIGHTING FAT

GET HIP WITH HEMP

Use hemp oil as a low-fat alternative to butter and vegetable oils in cooking. Not only is it low in fat, it's also high in omega-3 and omega-6 essential fatty acids (EFAs).

LOSE A BITTER FAT

Eating bitter orange, aka citrus aurantium, stimulates weight loss by increasing the production of heat to burn fat calories at a faster rate, giving the body access to greater amounts of energy.

KNOW YOUR NUMBERS

For every 10g of fat contained in a meal, women store nearly 4g in sub-cutaneous tissue (men store less than half this amount), so knowing how much fat is on your plate will help you work out how much exercise you will need to do to burn it off! The recommended daily fat intake for an average woman is 70g (2½oz).

DROP THE DRESSING TO DROP A DRESS SIZE

The average woman gets more fat from salad dressing than from any other food source. Just 2 tablespoons of salad dressing can contain between 10g and 20g of fat. To lighten up, try oil-free dressings or choose fat-free lemon juice instead.

COUNT ON CHROMIUM

Chromium helps control sugar cravings and suppress appetite, but many people's diets don't contain very much of this element because the natural soil reserves fresh produce is grown in are slowly being depleted; a supplement may help.

LINK STEAK AND SPINACH TO STAY LEAN

The amino acid L-carnitine, contained in lean meat, helps the body burn fat and it works even better when it's combined with vegetables such as spinach that contain another amino acid called lysine.

BURN FAT WHILE YOU REST

Exercising regularly helps boost your metabolism because muscle cells require more energy than fat cells in order to function. People who take regular exercise burn off about 600 more calories a week (and that is equivalent to the calories in four pieces of cheesecake!).

GIVE FAT THE COLD SHOULDER

A good and simple way to help your body fight fat is to drink ice-cold water. This causes more calories to be used up by the body than drinking water at room temperature because the digestive system has to use extra energy to heat it to body temperature.

FIX ON 45

If you are exercising at a steady pace, you need to keep going for more than 45 minutes before your body's potential for burning fat is optimal.

GO GREEN TO DROP WEIGHT

As well as containing metabolism-boosting caffeine, green tea has a secret ingredient with thermogenic properties. This means it increases energy production and stimulates fat oxidation in the body.

EAT APPLES TO FIGHT THE BULGE

The high levels of leptin in apples and celery help the body metabolize fat cells and reduce fat storage in subcutaneous layers, helping you stay smooth and slim.

A SEEDY WAY TO LOSE FAT

Eating some seeds instead of a high-fat snack could doubly boost weight loss by increasing your intake of leucine – found in soya, whey, nuts and seeds – which reduces body fat during weight loss.

COMBINE FOOD GROUPS

Pyruvate, a substance created in the body as it digests and metabolizes carbohydrates and proteins, has been shown to promote weight loss, so beware of faddy diets that separate carbs and proteins.

KEEP A DIARY

Keeping a food diary is a good method of cutting down on your calorie intake by making yourself aware of how much you really eat every day, and what your weaknesses are. Then rebalance your diet in favour of low-fat fruits, vegetables and complex carbohydrates.

BUILD MUSCLE TO BURN CALORIES AT REST

Muscle is the most metabolically active part of your body and burns up to three times as many calories as any other tissue. Add some resistance training to your workout to boost lean muscle and help you burn off calories in your downtime.

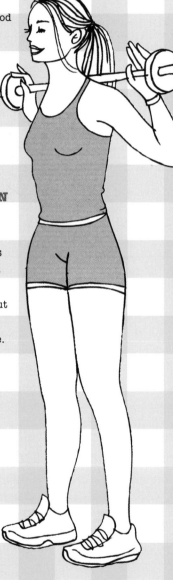

INDULGENCES

INDULGE YOUR SCENT-SES

Most of the tastes we love are strongly determined by our sense of smell. So the next time you desire a treat, try inhaling its aroma deeply instead of putting the item straight in your mouth. Often, the smell can be satisfying enough.

FEEL FULLER WITH NUTS

Recent research has found that eating a handful of peanuts every day can help you reduce your weight. This is because the peanuts produce a feeling of fullness, which, in turn, means you eat less later. The nuts also lower fat levels in the blood, which is good news for the heart.

MIRACLE FOODS

BUILD 24-CARROT BONES

If you want to build up the health of your bones without putting on any weight, then drink a glass of carrot juice every day. Carrot juice contains eight times as much calcium as milk, a host of other vitamins, and is packed with beneficial gut-regulating fibre.

GRAB A GRAPEFRUIT FOR WEIGHT LOSS

Eating grapefruit really does help people lose weight, and could reduce the risk of developing diabetes. Researchers have found that people who include grapefruit in their diet lose weight faster, an effect they think may be due to high levels of digestive enzymes in the fruit.

EAT YOURSELF HAPPY

Choose foods that are high in the mood-boosting substance tryptophan, including bananas, turkey, milk, yogurt, tuna and chicken, to help you stay happy and content between meals.

SALT

MAKE A HERBAL AGREEMENT

Instead of using salt, substitute herbs and spices, such as oregano, basil, coriander, thyme, parsley, cinnamon, nutmeg, cayenne pepper or paprika. Or season with lemon, garlic or vinegar.

GARGLE TO TARGET ULCERS

Saltwater can help prevent infection by clearing up damaging bacteria, particularly in sensitive areas. Studies have shown that gargling or mouthwashing with saltwater can significantly speed up the healing of mouth ulcers.

DETOX WITH A SALTY SPA

Detox skin and help yourself relax by adding half a cup of sea salt to your bath as it fills up. Not only will it stimulate your skin, you'll float better in it, taking the strain off muscles.

SALTY SCRUB FOR BETTER CIRCULATION

Mix 2 cups of fine sea salt with 4 cups of grapeseed, apricot or almond oil and 20 drops of your favourite essential oil. Vigorously but gently massage into damp skin, beginning at the feet, in a circular motion. Avoid any scratched or wounded areas. The scrub will help your circulation and improve the texture of the skin.

SUGAR & FATS

SHOW ME THE HONEY

Honey has fewer calories than sugar, it can help boost immunity and it is a good, natural alternative to refined sugars. If you're feeling under the weather, try manuka honey, made with pollen from the tea tree, famed for its healing powers.

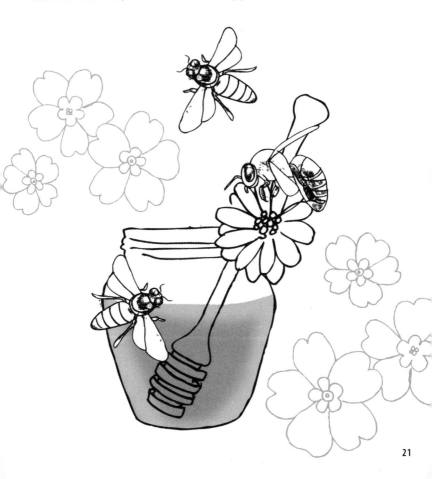

GO CANADIAN

Maple syrup is sweet and natural, with half the calories of normal sugar. For a healthy alternative to your usual sweetener, drizzle a few drops of maple syrup into tea or coffee or over desserts and discover its delicious and distinctive woody taste.

BEAT SUGAR FATIGUE

Fatigue could be due to fluctuations in blood sugar, which can cause metabolic changes in the body. Switch to slow-release sugars, such as fructose from fruit, to get your energy back.

EAT TO DRINK

Alcohol, especially if drunk with sugary mixer drinks, raises blood sugar and can lead to a blood sugar 'crash' later on, which is why people often feel hungry after a night out. The best foods to eat if you're hungry for a post-drink snack are ones that release energy slowly to regulate your blood sugar levels – oats, fruit, pasta and wholegrains.

DON'T FALL FOR THE FAT TRAP

Calories in the form of sugar are just as fattening as calories in the form of fat – all excess calories are stored in the body as fat tissue, so don't fall into the low-fat, high-sugar trap.

CAN THE FIZZ

Just one can of carbonated soda can contain up to 35g (1¼oz) of sugar, as much as several packets of sweets. So the next time you feel like something bubbly, try sparkling mineral water instead.

VITAMINS

FOCUS ON FOLATE

Folate is not only essential for all-over body health, it's also a key ingredient for foetal development in the first three months of pregnancy. Get your dose from mushrooms, bananas, egg yolks, lentils, beans, peanuts, fortified breads and cereals, leafy green vegetables, romaine lettuce, oranges and other citrus fruits and juices.

TAKE VITAMINS TO CATCH FREE RADICALS

Women need more antioxidants than men to mop up higher levels of free radicals and other negative elements in the female body. Vitamins C and E have been shown to maintain healthy arteries for heart health.

C OUT YOUR CENTURY

Vitamin C doesn't only reduce the risk of heart disease and other illness: it can also help you live longer. Studies have shown that people with high levels of vitamin C in their blood can increase the length of their life by several years.

PROTECT AGAINST MS

High levels of vitamin D could help protect you against the development of multiple sclerosis (MS), especially if it is taken in quantities of more than 400 IU (international units) a day, which could slash risk by up to a third. Vitamin D is also known to help the body absorb calcium, essential for strong bones.

BREATHE EASY WITH E, A AND C

Vitamins A, C and E are essential for the best lung functioning, especially in young men and women, so to ensure you breathe easy for life, top up on these health-giving vitamins, found in fresh fruits and vegetables, fruit juice and supplements.

SPRING CLEAN YOUR ARTERIES

Taking a supplement containing vitamins B12, B6 and folic acid could help prevent your arteries from getting blocked by lowering levels of artery-damaging homocysteine in the blood.

WEIGHT

DRINK UP TO FEEL FULL

Sipping water with food encourages the fibre in food to swell, making you feel fuller for longer. It also stimulates the liver to produce beneficial blood-cleaning fats, which moderate the rate and level at which your body absorbs fat and so help keep you looking slim.

BE WARY OF WOLFING

Instead of wolfing down meals and snacks, take time to savour them. People who spend more time and attention on eating tend to eat less and avoid overeating.

PLAY CHOPSTICKS

Using chopsticks or swapping your knife and fork into the wrong hands will make you work harder to get the food into your mouth, which uses up more calories. It may also encourage you to take smaller bites.

THINK OF THIRST FIRST

Feeling hungry? Make sure your body's not confusing thirst with hunger by drinking a glass of water before you start eating. Many of us have poor thirst mechanisms and may reach for food when we should be trying to get our optimum target of 2 litres (3½ pints) of water a day.

FIDGET AWAY FAT

Researchers believe extra movements burn up more calories. So in order to keep your body burning unwanted fat, always be on the move. Any extra body movements you can introduce into your normal day-to-day routine – from shifting your position more often than usual when sitting down, to occupying your hands when watching the television (whether you do this by playing with a stress-relieving toy or ironing the bed linen doesn't matter) will help you lose weight more easily. Try hiding the remote control (if you know where it is, of course) so you have to get up to change the channels or adjust the volume.

KEEP DRINKING TO DROP WEIGHT

If you don't seem to be able to lose weight, or your diet has stopped showing results, check how much water you've been drinking. Water levels need to be kept high to keep the metabolism rate at weight-loss potential.

DO YOUR MATHS

Weight loss is a simple maths formula: 450g (1lb) of weight is equal to 3,500 calories, so you need to cut back by about 500 calories a day to lose 450g (1lb) a week.

SLEEP YOURSELF SLIM

If you sleep for less than six hours a night, you could reduce your body's ability to burn off sugar, which means it is stored as fat instead. Make sure you sleep for seven to eight hours to stay slim.

FITNESS & WELLBEING

AROMATHERAPY

LIE DOWN WITH LAVENDER

Inhaling essential oil of lavender has been shown to have sedative and relaxing effects, so add a few drops to your pillow if you suffer from insomnia. It makes a perfect bedtime partner on hard-to-sleep nights.

PICK A PICK-ME-UP

The garden herbs basil and rosemary could mimic the effects of get-up-and-go hormones adrenaline and cortisol in the bloodstream, giving you extra energy to get through long days. Use them in cooking or use fresh or dried herbs to scent rooms.

SOAK AWAY YOUR BAD MOOD

Adding 3–5 drops of essential oil to a warm bath can either invigorate you or relax you, depending on the oil. Orange, grapefruit, ginger and peppermint are stimulating and will help you get going while lavender, geranium, rose and neroli are relaxing and calming.

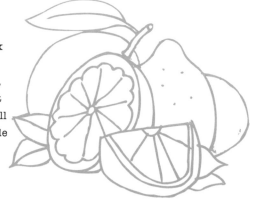

BALANCE

KEEP SKIN SILKY-SMOOTH
Exfoliating the skin to remove dead skin cells may help you retain
a good sense of balance by heightening the sensation powers of
your skin, thus allowing your body to make tiny adjustments.

GET FIT TO STAND TALL
Fitter people have better balance, not just because of their
tendency to be the correct weight but also because their nerves and
muscles are used to working together to keep their body upright.

BE A FLAMINGO FOR BETTER BALANCE
Practise standing on one leg, with your eyes fixed on a
stationary spot in front of you. Start on a hard floor and
progress to carpet or foam. Once you can stand balanced for a
whole minute, try changing the positions of your arms, legs and
eyes without falling over.

CIRCULATION

GET A SENSE OF HUMMUS
Increasing fibre intake helps level out circulation by aiding fluid
balance after eating. Pulse (legume) spreads like hummus and
bean dips, in place of sour cream and cheese spreads or dips, are
tasty ways to eat more fibre.

SPRINKLE AWAY STICKINESS

Vitamin E, which is found commonly in seeds like pumpkin and linseed (flax) and in fruits such as cherries, kiwi and green peppers, has been shown to reduce the stickiness of the blood, so reducing the possibility of clotting. Sprinkle the seeds on salads for a daily dose.

POUND AWAY PRESSURE

Working out at least three times a week boosts circulation, clears out arteries and lowers blood pressure, giving the circulation system an energy boost.

DETOX YOUR ARTERIES

Studies have shown that eating garlic can help reduce the buildup of plaque in arteries, and even clear away existing deposits. Aim to include some in your diet once a day or take a supplement.

CORE STRENGTH

HAVE A BALL

Swiss ball exercises can help strengthen your spine and core muscles safely and easily. Try swapping the sofa for a ball as you watch television, or engaging your body fully by using one at your work desk instead of a chair.

THINK YOURSELF STRONG

Hard to believe, but imagining yourself with strong core abdominal muscles could actually make them stronger by more than 10%. It's no substitute for exercise, but it's better than nothing!

BE STRAIGHT WITH YOURSELF

Try this simple exercise: stand up straight with your eyes closed
and concentrate on feeling the muscles in your body adapting to
keep you in position. This will help core strength as well as your
balance.

WORK IT AT WORK

Don't allow yourself to fall into bad habits at work that can ruin
your posture. For toning, and to remind yourself to stay strong
at the core, contract your abdominals and pelvic floor muscles
from time to time as you sit at your desk.

PULL IN YOUR BELLY TO PROTECT YOUR BACK

Having poor core strength makes you many times more susceptible
to injury and lower-back pain, as the spine is forced into adopting
unnatural positions. To support your lower back, pull your
bellybutton upwards and backwards until you feel 'lifted'.

ENERGY BOOSTERS

CRUNCH CRACKERS FOR GOOD SNACKING

Wholewheat or rice crackers spread with peanut butter, tahini,
hummus or low-fat savoury spreads like tapenade have been
shown to help weight loss and boost energy levels by curbing
unhealthy snacking.

HAVE A BRAZILIAN

No, not a bikini wax, but a healthy eating alternative instead!
Brazil nuts not only boost short-term energy, but just three a day
can also help cut the risk of heart disease by a third.

BE A SUNFLOWER SEEKER

Toasted sunflower seeds are a great choice to nibble on when afternoons at work begin to drag. Not only will they stop you reaching for fatty, salty snacks, they'll also boost your energy-giving vitamin levels while you munch.

APPRECIATE THE APRICOT

Dried apricots, perfect substitutes for biscuits (crackers) with cheese, are an excellent source of fibre, potassium, iron and betacarotene. Choose air-dried, not sulphur-dried, as sulphites have been linked to different forms of cancer.

STRETCH AND YAWN TO WORK OUT FACE MUSCLES

Stretching allows blood to flow into muscles that have become inactive, which is why it's so regenerating after sleep. Yawning gives your body a big oxygen boost, which combines with the stretching to give muscles instant energy.

FEEL CHIPPER WITH BANANA

For a handy and tasty pick-me-up, why not try dried banana chips? They are rich in carbohydrates, iron and magnesium and, in addition, they have natural sugars to give your body an energy boost when you're on the move. Combine them with plain, natural yogurt when you're looking for a more substantial snack.

WAKE UP TO MORNING GLORY

For a morning boost, swap your first cup of tea or coffee for an energy-giving detox drink made with hot water, lemon juice, freshly grated ginger, maple syrup and a pinch of cayenne pepper.

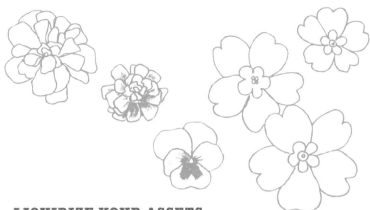

LIQUIDIZE YOUR ASSETS

Make a natural power drink by liquidizing apples, banana and
a tablespoon of peanut butter together. Drink a glass with your
breakfast. The fruit sugars will boost your energy at different
levels to keep you going all morning.

FEEL BLOOMING GOOD

Add a ray of natural sunshine to your life by feasting on edible
flowers like violets, nasturtiums, marigolds, primroses and
pansies, which can benefit body and mind.

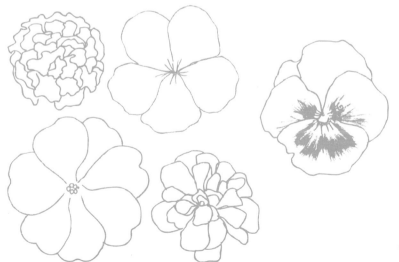

EYESIGHT

KEEP AGEING EYES IN THE CAN

Eating canned tuna more than once a week reduces the risk of developing age-related macular degeneration by more than 40%. Combine with vitamin-rich sweet potato and tomato for the best benefits.

TREAT YOURSELF TO A BERRY GOOD VIEW

Compounds called flavonoids, found in berries, protect the sensitive cells of the eye, which are especially prone to strain from work at computers. Drink a blueberry smoothie for a bright-eyed day.

LOOK YOURSELF IN THE EYES

If the whites of your eyes appear dull or yellowish in colour, this could be an indication of a struggling liver. Help it out with milk thistle, ginger and citrus fruits.

FOCUS ON FISH

Omega-3 fish oils are thought to protect the macula lutea (the spot at the centre of the retina) from problems. Aim to eat oily fish like tuna, mackerel or salmon more than once a week and use linseed (flaxseed) and sunflower oils for cooking.

EAT SWEET POTATO FOR SWEET VISION

Although they taste rich and creamy, sweet potatoes are fat- and cholesterol-free and full of vision-boosting betacarotene and vitamin A. One medium-sized sweet potato has only around 130 calories.

CHOCOLATE FOR FIRST-RATE VISION

A daily dose of chocolate, particularly the dark, high cocoa-solids varieties, can help vision by topping up copper levels.

CUT OUT WHEAT AND BANISH UNDEREYE CIRCLES

Dark circles under the eyes, usually considered a sign of tiredness, can also be caused by food intolerance, often to refined foods. Try cutting out processed foods for a few days and see if they lighten up.

GIVE YOUR EYES A REST

Even if you have only a minute to spare, focus on something far away, blink several times to build up moisture, then hold the lids closed for a few seconds, pressing your palms over the sockets to rest and rejuvenate the eyes.

FERTILITY

COUNT TEN TO CONCEPTION

Women wishing to conceive should make love every other day for a ten-day period during the middle of their cycle. Studies have shown that the five days before and the five days after the projected ovulation date are the most promising times to become pregnant.

RAISE A CUP TO FERTILI-TEA

Taking an infusion from 125g (4oz) or more of tea each day could double, or even in some cases triple, your chances of conception. Black teas contain slightly more caffeine than green, but either will do the trick.

DON'T BE A LEMON

Calming coffee-free drinks like hot water with lemon juice may actually harm chances of conception because lemon juice has been shown to kill sperm, not only directly but also by altering the acid levels in the body.

IMMUNITY BOOSTS

GRAB A GRAPE

Grapes, especially those with seeds, could boost immunity by inducing the production of important cells known as T-cells, which play a key part in protecting against viruses and bacteria in the body.

SHORT-TERM BOOSTS

Echinacea – available as tablets or a liquid – stimulates phagocytosis, the consumption of invading organisms by white blood cells. The herb has maximum effect when taken in short courses to fight recurring infections, such as colds. For this reason, avoid taking it as a long-term preventive measure.

POSTURE

DON'T LET SHOULDERS CREEP UP ON YOU

A common fault is to let shoulders creep up towards your ears as muscles tighten and the back bends forward. Gently hold shoulders back and try to keep space around the sides of your neck.

WALK TALL TO FREE YOUR BACK

As you walk around, lift your head until you're looking straight ahead of you, with a relaxed neck and shoulders. Press your shoulders back (not up) so your chest is pushed out, and straighten your spine so you are standing straight, but not too rigidly, like a ramrod.

KEEP CIRCULATION HEALTHY WITH THE THREE-FINGER GAP

If your feet are hanging or tucked under when you sit down, the increased pressure on the backs of the legs can impair return circulation from the feet. This can lead to or aggravate swollen ankles and varicose veins. Keep both feet on the floor and aim for no more than a a three-finger gap behind your knees.

GET FIRM AT NIGHT

Make sure your mattress is firm enough to support the contours of your body, to reduce pressure on the spine.

PULL YOUR KEYBOARD CLOSER

By holding your elbows away from your body you set up continuous tension in the muscles of the neck and shoulders, thus creating a buildup of lactic acid and other unwelcome by-products. If you're typing, make sure the keyboard is positioned so that your elbows fall to your sides, not in front of you.

WALK FASTER, NOT LONGER

It is counterproductive – and potentially harmful to your back – to increase the length of your stride unnaturally. Speed and efficiency in walking are generated by hip flexibility and using quicker, not longer, steps.

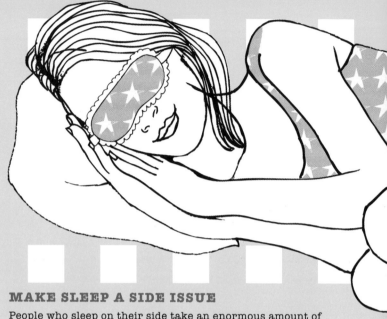

MAKE SLEEP A SIDE ISSUE

People who sleep on their side take an enormous amount of pressure off their spine compared with those who lie on their front or back. Lying face down is the worst position for overnight spine health.

GIVE IT THE ELBOW

By bending your arms at the elbow when you walk, and using them to work your stride pattern, you will burn at least 5%-10% more calories than if you let them hang by your side.

SLEEPING SUPPORT

If you lie on your side in bed at night, consider putting a pillow between your knees to keep them at the same width as your hips, and so reduce twisting and strain on the pelvis. This will also help you avoid the discomfort of hip pain.

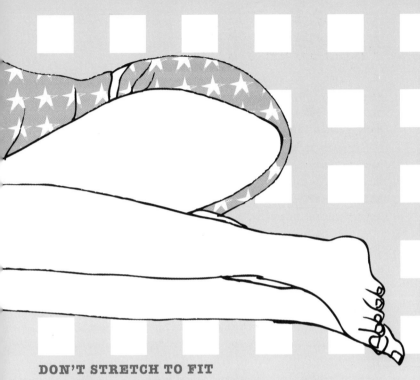

DON'T STRETCH TO FIT

For perfect posture, your neck should not be straight or stretched, but it should retain its slight natural curve with your chin parallel to the floor, neither tucked in nor jutting out.

IMAGINE A GOLDEN STRING
TO BETTER POSTURE

This health tip is borrowed from the Alexander Technique, and it is a way to help you walk taller without injury. Imagine there is a golden string running vertically up your body through your spine, stretching you upwards through the crown of your head and creating space between each vertebra.

PRESSURE POINTS

GIVE YOURSELF A HELPING HAND

Your LI4 pressure point is located on the top side of the hand, between your thumb and your index finger. To locate it, squeeze the thumb against the base of the index finger. The point you are looking for is located on the highest point of the bulge of the muscle. Press this point for about 30 seconds to induce calmness and for a health-inducing digestive detox. However, you should not try this technique if you are pregnant.

PUT YOUR BEST FOOT FORWARD

Your L3 pressure point is found on the foot, on the line running between the big toe and the second toe and about three finger widths from the edge in the hollow on the top of the foot. Move your index finger anticlockwise over this point in order to induce relaxation and to unblock any anger and depression.

COMPRESS THE WRIST TO REDUCE
THE STRESS

Find the spot between the tendons of the inside of the wrist, three finger widths from the palm. Breathe in, press as you breathe out slowly and repeat several times to reduce stress and strain.

CLEAR YOUR KIDNEYS

Your kidney point, which can be used to treat fatigue and lethargy as well as to detox the body through the kidneys, is located on the sole of the foot, just to the side of the ball of the foot under the second or third toe. Press and release several times.

ENJOY AN EXTRA ENERGY BOOST

Stimulating your stomach point can give you extra energy when you're flagging or tired. It is located just below the knee, on the outside of the shinbone. Press for at least 30 seconds with the pad of your finger or thumb.

TEND TO NECK TENSION

A tension-relief point, good for reducing pain caused by tension headaches and relieving tired eyes, is found in the occipital hollow, where the bottom of the skull meets the neck on either side of the spine. Use a thumb on either side to compress this area but be very careful not to press too hard.

ARM YOURSELF AGAINST ANXIETY

A stress-relieving point for reducing anxiety and tension is found at the top centre of the forearm (with palm facing down) in the large section of muscle just underneath the crease of the elbow. Press for several seconds and release several times.

LISTEN TO YOUR HEART

Your SI19 point is located near the ear, just before the small projection in front of the ear canal. It's in the depression that forms when the mouth is opened. Press for several seconds to release your inner emotions and desires.

STEP UP TO BOOST METABOLISM

A metabolism-boosting point is found on top of the foot, roughly in line with the middle two toes and directly over the arch. Use two fingers to apply broader pressure here because of the bones and ligaments.

GET IMMEDIATE IMMUNITY

An immunity-boosting point that is also good for combating fatigue, depression and general feelings of sluggishness is found on the inside of the ankle above the foot between the Achilles tendon and the ankle bone. Press and release several times for 10–20 seconds.

FORM A FIST TO HELP A HEADACHE

A point for general pain relief (especially of headaches) is found on the back, in line with the kidneys. The best way to stimulate this point is to sit up straight on a chair and form a fist with both hands. Place the fists behind your back so they touch and lie level with the elbow. Lean back gently.

DO AN ANTISTRESS PRESS

Stimulating the acupressure point that is located in the soft V-shaped area of flesh found between the thumb and forefinger can help reduce stress. Press the pad of your thumb into this area for at least 30 seconds and then repeat the same action on the other hand.

SELF-MASSAGE

GET IT OFF YOUR CHEST

In order to reduce tension across the front of the chest area, and to free up your breathing and loosen stress in your neck, place the four fingers of your right hand on the left side of your chest, underneath the clavicle bone. Move the fingers in circular motions, working outward towards the shoulder joint in deeper strokes. Repeat on the other side. Breathe in and out slowly as you massage.

HEAD OFF TENSION
To reduce tension in the scalp, spread out the fingers and thumbs of both hands and place them on either side of your head with the thumbs towards the back of the neck. Work in small circular motions, and then, after a few seconds, move the hands so they cover a different area.

STICK YOUR NECK OUT
To reduce neck tension, move the four fingers of your right hand in circular motions over the top of your left shoulder, turning your head to the right to stretch the muscles and ligaments at the front of the neck. Repeat on the other side.

DRAW TENSION FROM YOUR JAW
To relieve tension in your jaw and the sides of your face, place the four fingers of your left hand together on the jaw so the index finger fits into the bony area in front of the earlobe. Using small circular motions, work lightly, being careful not to press too hard.

SENSE & SENSATION

EAT BEFORE YOU GET TOO HUNGRY
Hungry people taste salt and sugar more strongly than people who aren't hungry, so to avoid those salt and sugar cravings don't go for long periods without eating – have a healthy snack before you feel ravenous.

SLEEP

HOLD YOUR TONGUE

Experts suggest that you try this clever sleep trick to help you drop off: close your eyes and hold your tongue so it's not touching your cheeks or the roof of your mouth, as if you're yawning with your mouth closed. You'll be sleeping like a log in no time.

BE A HERBAL HIBERNATOR

Certain herbs such as valerian, camomile, hops and lime tree flowers have been shown to have sedative properties and are often taken either internally as a herbal tea or used within herbal pillows to enhance sleep.

BEAT SNORING BY SLEEPING MORE

Sleep deprivation, especially if it's over several weeks, causes the muscles of the throat to sag, which leads to more snoring and less sleep. To stop snoring, aim for at least seven hours of sleep a night.

DON'T EXERCISE LAST THING AT NIGHT

Because undertaking physical exercise raises internal body temperature, which, in turn, wakes you up, exercising before bedtime is not a good way to tackle insomnia. Instead, try relaxing stretches or an indulgent bath.

KEEP YOUR SLEEP ON SCHEDULE

According to the experts, going to sleep at about the same time every night helps your body get into a regular sleep rhythm, which will help put a stop to any sleep problems. Similarly, try to get up at the same time every day in order to keep your schedule on track.

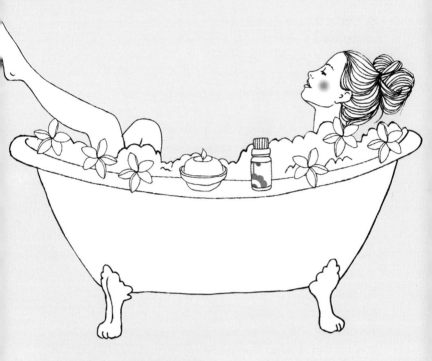

SOAK AWAY INSOMNIA

A warm bath before bedtime can help you sleep by relaxing
muscles and encouraging inactivity, which is essential for sleep.
Try using calming aromatherapy oils such as lavender and
lowering the lighting for an even sleepier experience.

PUT SLEEP FIRST

Lack of sleep impairs your coordination, judgement and immune
system, say the experts, so put sleep first for a healthy life and
get into good habits by going to bed at about the same time every
night. If a particular job or task isn't done by bedtime, just leave
it until tomorrow.

AVOID CAFFEINE AFTER DARK

Caffeine has well-known stimulant effects and drinking it before bed is likely to impair the quality of your sleep. Remember that chocolate contains caffeine, too, so that late-night treat might not in reality be a good idea either.

AIR YOUR SHEETS TO REFRESH YOUR SLEEP

Bacteria, mites and bedbugs thrive in moist conditions; so after you get up in the morning and instead of making the bed immediately, turn back the covers to allow the sheets to breathe for 30 minutes. Airing your bedroom by opening a window will help, too.

WORKOUT WISDOM

DRINK UP TO WORK OUT

Because water is essential to maximize metabolism, you won't reap the full benefits from your exercise routine unless you stay hydrated throughout. You can boost your body's performance on workouts simply by keeping topped up with water. Studies have shown that just a 3% loss in body fluid can lead to a 7% reduction in overall physical performance; so drink plenty of water before, during and after your workouts.

GET INTENSE

High-intensity workouts have a greater and longer-lasting effect on increasing your resting metabolic rate, essential for long-term fat burning. Researchers have found that upping the intensity when you work out could help you burn as much as 300 extra calories a day, even at rest.

DO EXERCISE TO AVOID DIABETES

Exercise reduces fat tissue in the body and makes cells more responsive to insulin. Exercising five times a week has been shown to reduce the risk of diabetes by 45%, two to four times a week by 40% and once a week by 25%.

BREATHE IN, BREATHE OUT

Keep breath flow steady to nourish your body with oxygen. As a rule, inhale on the easy part of an exercise and exhale on the hard part to keep optimum oxygen levels.

STEP IT UP IN STYLE

Don't crank up the resistance on the Stairmaster or step machine so high that you have to lean on the arm posts, because this reduces efficiency. Instead, pump with your legs, get your heart rate up and progress slowly as you feel more comfortable with each level.

SCORE A GOAL OF THE MONTH

Set small, realistic goals – don't set yourself up for failure by aiming for unachievable targets. Decide on small goals you can achieve, such as three 30-minute sessions at the gym each week, which make it easier to experience success.

GIVE YOURSELF A GOLD MEDAL

Reward yourself for your successes. When you don't feel like exercising, remember how good you felt after exercising the last time, and reward yourself with healthy treats such as exercise clothes, new music to work out to or a sports massage.

BE A VARIETY PERFORMER

For most of us, doing the same workout routine daily can induce boredom, not only in your head but also in your body, as it adapts to tasks. So vary your workouts and type of exercise to boost mental and physical fitness.

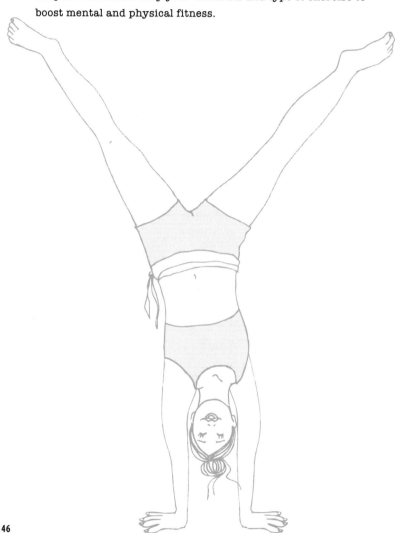

PUT YOUR BACK INTO IT

When devising a complete exercise plan, don't forget back exercises – although they might not seem as important as those showy triceps curls or leg squats, a strong back is absolutely key to effective, injury-free training.

POSTURE-PERFECT WORKOUTS

As you work out, don't forget to engage your core strength muscles in your abdomen, which will keep your trunk strong and steady and help you avoid succumbing to injury, as well as preventing bad exercise habits.

DON'T CURL UP TO SIT UP

Many people don't really work their abdominals properly during their situp exercise routines. Make sure you are moving the top of your body towards the ceiling, rather than curling it up towards your knees, which doesn't work the muscles as hard.

ANYONE FOR TENNIS?

Tennis burns 400 calories an hour and although it might not be such a good cardio-vascular exercise as running or swimming, the tactical thinking stimulates your mind as well as your body, giving you a true holistic workout.

SQUASH UP YOUR BACKSIDE

Played competitively, squash will really firm up your arms and abdominals, as well as giving your system a cardiovascular boost. But it is also one of the best exercises around for toning up those flabby behinds because of all the lunging around court that is involved.

SADDLE UP TO RIDE AWAY SADDLE BAGS

Horse-riding not only tones hips, legs and thighs through a series of leg exercises as you ride, it also increases strength and flexibility in your pelvis, hips and lower back, and works the thigh muscles to reduce fat.

BOULDER YOUR WAY TO BETTER ARMS

If rock climbing is perhaps just a bit too extreme for you but you'd love the upper-body benefits, then try the safer alternative of bouldering. This is a sport in which you travel along the rockface rather than scaling it upwards. It builds great arm strength and, as a bonus, burns a whopping 360 calories in just 30 minutes.

BOWL AWAY CALORIES

Next time you're playing a game of baseball, softball, rounders or cricket, volunteer to bowl or pitch – it burns the most calories of any other position on the playing field.

PUNCH YOUR FIGHTS OUT

For the ultimate body- and brain-boosting workout, invest in a punchbag and a skipping rope. It has been shown that working out like a boxer will not only increase your cardiovascular fitness but also get rid of aggression and allow stress to flow out of the system.

WORKOUT BURNOUT

Overtraining can be just as dangerous as under-training. To prevent problems, make sure you have at least one complete rest day a week and give yourself a whole week off every two to three months to stay physically and mentally healthy.

BOOST METABOLISM BY WORKING OUT EARLY

A workout first thing in the morning helps fire the metabolism all day, and when your metabolism is higher, you burn more calories. As a consequence, morning workouts mean you can eat the same amount and still lose weight.

BE STRETCH EFFECTIVE

Stretches are ineffective unless they are held for a certain time. You should ease into position until you feel the stretch, then hold it for at least 25 seconds. Breathe deeply to help your body move oxygen-rich blood to sore muscles.

GET RID OF YOUR JELLY BELLY

Belly dancing, because of its constant use of the abdominal and pelvic muscles, is one of the best exercises you can choose to tone up flabby bellies. It's fun, social and sexy, too – what more could you ask of a workout?

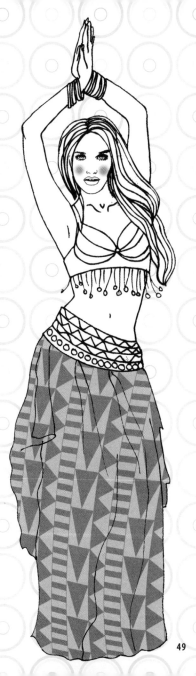

ILLNESS & AILMENTS

ALLERGIES

STAY IN TO DRY OUT

To avoid windborne pollen and grass seeds coming into contact
with you, sticking to your clothes and causing allergic reactions,
dry clothes and bedding inside instead of hanging them out on
a clothesline.

BRING BACK BATHTIME

Remember when the last thing you did before bed was have a
bath? Washing your skin and hair in the evening rather than
in the morning has been shown to reduce allergic reactions
overnight by getting rid of allergens in hair and on skin.

A SWEET HEALER

The healing properties of honey are thought to flow from its high
proportions of pollen and plant compounds, producing a natural
immunity in the body. Bee pollen, royal jelly, honeycomb and
unfiltered honey are all believed to help.

C FOR YOURSELF

Vitamin C is definitely the wonder vitamin when it comes to
your immune system. Make sure you get a generous daily dose
of fresh fruit and vegetables or take a supplement to keep your
body fit to fight off infections.

GET STEAMY TO CLEAR YOUR HEAD

Coughing during the night can be eased by hanging a wet towel on or near a radiator to increase humidity in the room overnight, preventing the lungs and throat from drying out and decreasing the chances of damage or infection.

GET SALTY FOR SINUSES

If your sinuses are causing problems, you might want to try the 3,000-year-old yogic practice of sniffing saltwater, which can help fight and prevent sinus infections. Ask a doctor or nurse for advice.

ARTHRITUS

GO ALKALINE TO NEUTRALIZE ACID PAIN

Acidic foods like tomato, citrus fruits, fruit juices and red meats can make the pain of arthritis worse by building up acid crystals in the joints. Instead, plump for high-alkaline or neutral foods like green vegetables, eggs, dairy produce and water.

EASE PAIN WITH PINEAPPLE

Pineapple has been shown to suppress inflammation and boost bone health, thus improving joint pain in arthritis. Its anti-inflammatory properties are thought to be due to its high bromelain content.

CURRY FLAVOUR TO STOP SWELLING

Curries that contain high levels of the herb turmeric contain circumin, a natural anti-inflammatory that can help alleviate pain and swelling. If you don't fancy the hot stuff, supplements are also available.

SOAK AWAY PAIN

Morning baths in warm water, or soaks for feet and hands, can help ease pain from arthritic joints, which is often worse first thing. Soak for at least ten minutes to reap maximum benefits.

TAKE UP TAI CHI FOR FLEXIBILITY

The ancient Chinese art of Tai Chi has been shown to reduce both the effects of arthritis and the distress caused by stiff, painful joints. Practising at least two or three times a week is most beneficial.

DROP A SIZE TO BE KNEE-WISE

According to experts, being overweight is such a danger to joints that losing as little as 5kg (11lb) may cut the risk of osteoarthritis of the knee by 50%.

RUE THE RHUBARB

Rhubarb contains oxalic acid, which inhibits your body's ability to absorb calcium and iron from other foods. It can aggravate arthritis and may even cause an attack if eaten to excess.

BE SUPER-CAREFUL IN THE SUN

Arthritis can make the skin more sensitive to the sun, so make sure you cover head, shoulders and eyes on bright days.

BACK PAIN

QUICK-RELEASE YOUR BACK

For a quick back stretch at your desk, place your feet flat on the ground and lean back on your chair so your back arches slightly. Drop your head backwards and then take a few deep breaths.

DESTRESS TO HELP YOUR BACK

Stress causes muscle tension that can lead to pain, especially in the lower back as the postural support muscles are overworked. Experts estimate that almost a fifth of all back pain is due to stress, so relaxation could be the most important prevention.

DON'T BE AN ARCH VILLAIN

The spine begins to show signs of wear and tear as early as age 35, so from this age onwards it's important to keep it flexible and strong. Lots of people forget that the back doesn't only bend forward – it's important to stretch it into an arched position as well. You can do this by simply leaning backwards to release muscles or try backwards bend yoga postures.

BAG A HEALTHY BACK

Carrying your bag on the same shoulder all the time can lead to muscle imbalance and weakness, leading to pain. Resolve to swap shoulders every other day or use a backpack.

BED DOWN IN COMFORT

Sleeping on your stomach can put the back and neck into various strained positions, causing stiffness and pain when you wake in the morning. To prevent problems developing, lie flat on your back with a pillow under your knees. Or sleep on your side with knees slightly bent and a pillow between your legs.

LOSE WEIGHT TO LESSEN PAIN

Being overweight forces your body to carry more than its natural weight and, as most people walk at least a mile every day just in normal life, every pound counts. Slimming down could help most overweight people with back problems.

SIT UP WITH SIT-UPS

It is estimated that strengthening the abdominal muscles could prevent more than 75% of lower-back problems. Regular sit-ups and abdominal exercises can help, as can core strength training with Pilates and yoga classes.

GIVE YOUR BACK SOME BACK-UP

Use a chair with a proper backrest to prevent pressure on the lower back, or slip a thin cushion or rolled-up jumper (sweater) behind your lower back for correct support.

BE A SCREEN SIREN

Make sure your computer screen is at the right height for comfortable viewing – you shouldn't need to lean towards or away from your screen, for example, and it should be level with your eyes. In addition, your arms should rest lightly on the desk's surface as you use the keyboard.

MAKE LIKE A CAT TO STRETCH YOUR BACK

To ease the strain and any discomfort in your back, get down on your hands and knees, hands palm down in line with shoulders, looking at the floor. Slowly push your back up into an upward curve, hold this for five seconds and then release. Repeat this ten times.

TILT YOUR PELVIS TO TREAT YOUR BACK

Try this pelvic exercise to ease any stress you might be feeling in the lower back region. Lie flat on your back with your legs bent and feet flat on the floor. Press your lower back to the floor by tightening the abdominal muscles; hold for ten seconds and then release the position. Repeat five times, breathing normally throughout.

SWIM INTO HEALTH

Swimming is an excellent exercise for healthy backs because it avoids the strain of impact sports and allows the body to realign itself while supported by the water.

PACK SOME HEAT TO DULL PAIN

To relieve chronic pain and stiffness in your back, try heated water therapies such as swimming pools, whirlpools, warm showers and steam rooms. Alternatively, apply warm compresses, hot towels or microwaveable heat packs to the area.

TOP UP ON CALCIUM

Calcium is essential for keeping the bones of the spine firm and flexible. There are plenty of sources besides milk, including yogurt, broccoli, kale, figs, almonds and calcium supplements.

BEATING CANCER

SWEAT IT AWAY

Studies have shown that regular physical exercise prompts a series of changes within the body that actively fight cancer. The risk of colon, breast, prostate and other cancers lessens with regular activity.

SPROUT A DOUBLE CANCER CURE

Green leafy vegetables contain a combination of two components that are 13 times more powerful at fighting cancer together than alone. Selenium and sulphoraphane are found in high levels in Brussels sprouts, broccoli and cabbage.

COUNT CALCIUM TO FIGHT CANCER

Low-fat diets that limit intake of dairy products could be exposing slimmers to colon cancer by reducing their calcium intake to dangerously low levels. Studies suggest that even small increases in calcium can cut the risk by half.

GO GREEN TO PROTECT YOURSELF

The polyphenols and catechins in green tea have powerful antioxidative and anticancer effects when taken regularly. Aim for at least one cup a day.

PEACHY KEEN

Peaches, sweet potatoes and apricots contain high levels of betacarotene, which cannot only prevent cancer cells from growing but can even kill them off.

UNDERCOOK FOR GOOD HEALTH

Charring food during roasting, grilling and barbecueing can produce carcinogens in the burned areas. The healthiest food is cooked through but not burned.

BE A GOOD BEAN

Eating beans, including chickpeas, kidney beans and lentils, on a regular basis – say, one portion every week – could cut the risk of death from cancer by nearly half. This is because beans contain various anticancer agents.

TRAIN YOUR TASTEBUDS

Sugar is a major risk factor for cancer. Instead of choosing high-sugar options, train your tastebuds by gradually reducing sugar in your diet or swapping it for healthy alternatives, such as apple juice, date sugar and rice syrup.

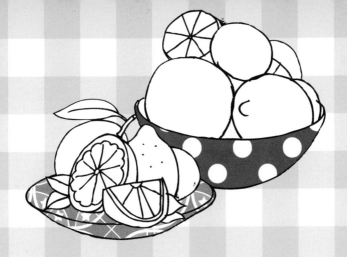

BE A LEMON TO FIGHT DISEASE

Citrus fruits, such as grapefruit, lemon and orange, are powerful anticancer agents because they contain a collection of all the natural substances known to ward off cancer cells.

BREATHING PROBLEMS

TALK THE TALK

A good way to keep your breathing calm and regular is to have a conversation with someone or to read out loud. Speech naturally regulates breathing, thus putting a stop to the short and shallow breaths that can lead to problems.

TAKE A DEEP BREATH

Taking a few deep breaths really does help you stay calm and in control, by stopping the release of the stress hormones adrenaline and cortisol into the blood.

STRIKE A POSE

Yoga has been shown to help breathing problems and asthma by reducing tension in the breathing muscles and expanding the ribs to allow more air inside the lungs. Aim for three sessions a week to reap the health rewards.

VITALIZE LUNGS WITH VITAMINS

A lack of vitamins C and E, betacarotene and selenium (found in lentils, avocados and brazil nuts) in the diet can harm the lungs so much that it's the equivalent of smoking a pack of 20 cigarettes a day for ten years.

EAT ONION TO PREVENT CANCER

Eating lots of onion, apple and yellow grapefruit regularly could help protect your body against developing lung cancer by destroying squamous cell carcinoma, which is a specific type of the disease. Combine cooked onion with raw apple and grapefruit for the most potent anticancer effect.

COLDS & FLU

THINK ZINC FOR SORE THROATS

Zinc gluconate lozenges may shorten colds by an average of three days as well as alleviate sore throats, nasal congestion, coughing, headaches and hoarseness.

SNIFF AWAY SYMPTOMS

Aromatherapy oils of black pepper, eucalyptus, hyssop, pine and sweet thyme can help get rid of coughs, colds and symptoms of congestion. Use with steam to alleviate symptoms further.

DON'T OVERLOAD ON WATER

Many people's first reaction when they come down with a respiratory infection is to drink copious amounts of water. However, some experts now believe that overdrinking could worsen the problem by leading to salt loss and fluid overload. Aim for 2 litres (3½ pints) a day.

STEAM-CLEAN YOUR NOSE

The steam from boiling water can help your system fight off infections, possibly by killing any viruses that have newly alighted in the mucous membranes of your nose. To stay healthy, get down to your local sauna or steam room or invest in a facial steamer for home use.

FEVER

CUT OUT MEAT TO CUT THE HEAT

Reducing iron if you have a temperature could help fight infection, so avoid iron-rich foods until you're on the mend, then stock up your levels as you recover.

MAKE YOUR TEMPERATURE TEPID

To ease the discomfort of a fever, don't use cold water, which can shock the skin into holding onto heat. Instead, get into a bath that feels the same as body temperature or dab yourself with a tepid flannel.

FIRST AID

SAY ALOE TO CALMER SKIN

Aloe vera has soothing properties that stop the inflammation and redness of skin rashes, including prickly heat. Apply liberally for best results.

BE INFECTION-FREE WITH TEA TREE

Cleansing, antiseptic tea tree oil can be applied directly to skin in order to help keep minor scrapes and wounds clean, and it has been shown to be a more powerful antibiotic than many modern drugs. Keep some handy in your medicine cabinet for day-to-day use.

A NATURAL ALTERNATIVE TO ANTIBIOTICS

Eucalyptus oil has long been prized for its healing abilities, but recent research studies have shown that it can be even more effective at fighting bacterial infections than some antibiotics.

KEEP BERRY COOL

On hot summer days, when heat-stroke is a possible hazard, enhance the body's natural cooling system with infusions of raspberry and peppermint tea.

FIGHT BITES WITH CITRONELLA

The aromas of tea tree, eucalyptus and citronella have been shown to repel mosquitoes and other biting insects, so apply the oils to exposed areas of the skin to ensure you don't get bitten.

HEADACHES

HOOK A HEADACHE CURE

Omega-3 essential fatty acids (EFAs), found in oily fish such as tuna and salmon, can lower the production of hormones that cause inflammation and pain, so eating fish regularly could help stop those migraines once and for all.

WATER DOWN THE TENDERNESS

Give yourself a pain-relieving massage by standing in the shower with the water stream directed to the back of your neck, then slowly turning to look behind you. This removes lactic acid from the muscles and makes the blood vessels less 'irritable'.

BITE THE BULLET

Poor tooth or jaw alignment has been found to be the cause of some chronic headaches. A few sessions in the dentist's chair could clear your head for good.

PAIN BETWEEN THE EYES

Less than perfect eyesight can trigger headaches because the eye and other muscles squeeze in order to focus. If your headaches come on after reading or working at a computer screen, make sure you give your eyes a rest every ten minutes by focusing on a distant object for at least 60 seconds. Make a point of having regular eye examinations, too.

INDULGE IN A SPOT OF COFFEE THERAPY

Coffee can help cure headaches because of the injection of caffeine it gives the body (but take care not to overdo the caffeine – many over-the-counter headache remedies already contain a healing dose).

SNIFF AN APPLE A DAY

Apples could keep the doctor away after all. Research studies have shown that the scent of green apples can reduce the severity of migraines, so the next time you feel a headache coming on, reach for the fruit bowl and inhale deeply.

HEART DISEASE

SAY ALOE TO A HEALTHY HEART

A diet that is supplemented with aloe vera and psyllium husks could set you on the road to having better heart health by reducing the amount of cholesterol in your system and improving the balance of good and bad cholesterol.

EARN SOME FAT PROFITS

Not all fat is bad. Beneficial essential fatty acids (EFAs), such as the omega-3 type found in fish, olives and flaxseed, have been shown to reduce the risk of heart disease. Instead of banning fat entirely from your diet, substitute good fats for the heart-harming trans fats found in many margarines, cooking oils and processed foods.

STEER CLEAR OF HYDROGENATED OILS

Just a few grams of omega-3 fatty acids a day can prevent
an irregular heart beat, decrease inflammation and promote
blood flow. Choose olive oil and fish oils instead of cooking oils,
because the hydrogenation process they go through destroys
omega-3.

JOINT PROBLEMS

GIVE BONES A D-DAY

Calcium isn't all we need to keep bones healthy and strong and
guard against osteoporosis as we get older. Studies have shown
that vitamin D in association with calcium boosts the body's
ability to make the most of both substances to increase bone
health and strength.

GALVANIZE SORE JOINTS WITH GLUCOSAMINE

Truly the wonder drug where the body's joints are concerned,
glucosamine occurs naturally in the body. In studies it has
been shown, time after time, to strengthen joints, reduce pain,
prevent injury and help protect against the degeneration that
comes with ageing. Glucosamine is even more effective when
taken with chondroitin, a closely related substance that prevents
body enzymes from degrading joint cartilage.

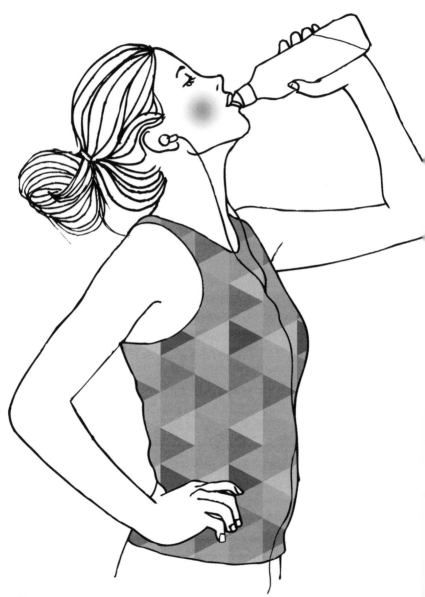

MUSCLE SORENESS

DRINK UP TO STOP STIFFNESS
Dehydration is a major cause of post-exercise muscle soreness.
Drinking water regularly while you work out should be sufficient
to keep levels high enough to combat pain.

REDUCE PAIN WITH VITAMIN C
Vitamin C and bioflavonoids may help offset the damage
that muscles endure during exercise. Taken regularly, these
nutrients reduce the incidence of sports injuries and shorten the
time it takes to recover from a muscle injury.

A PINEAPPLE PICK-UP
Bromelain, which is a fruit extract taken from the pineapple, has
potent anti-inflammatory properties in the body that can help to
reduce muscle soreness brought about by inflammation. And the
fruit gives you a good dose of vitamins that help healing, too.

DRINK SMOOTHIES TO HEAL MUSCLE TEARS
Combine calcium-rich milk with potassium-packed banana for a
smoothie to treat muscles cramps and soreness after exercise.
Calcium and potassium help muscles heal microtears that can
cause pain.

NAUSEA

ROOT OUT SICKNESS

Ginger root, taken as powder or tea, works directly in the gastrointestinal tract by interfering with the feedback mechanisms that send sickness messages to the brain.

PRESS AWAY DISCOMFORT

Acupressure wristbands, which attach around the forearm and press against certain antisickness acupressure points, have been shown to help prevent motion sickness and nausea.

BECOME AN OLD SOAK

Soaking beans in water can help turn their indigestible, wind- and nausea-inducing components into easier-to-digest substances. For the best results, soak them thoroughly and change the water at least once while cooking them.

FIBRE PROVIDERS

For a healthy digestive system, we should aim for an intake of around 20–35g (1–1½oz) of fibre a day, which is equivalent to a couple of pieces of wholemeal bread or a bowl of muesli. Other good dietary sources are vegetables and oats.

DON'T DO FAST FOOD

Meals that are eaten in front of the television, at your desk or on the move are more likely to cause nausea and sickness. As an alternative, give yourself some quiet time in a comfortable seat to enjoy chewing and tasting every morsel of your slow food.

PRESS YOUR ANTISICKNESS BUTTON

The acupressure point P6 is thought to relieve nausea and travel sickness. It is located between the tendons on the inside arm, three finger widths above the wrist crease. Press lightly for 30 seconds whenever you need relief.

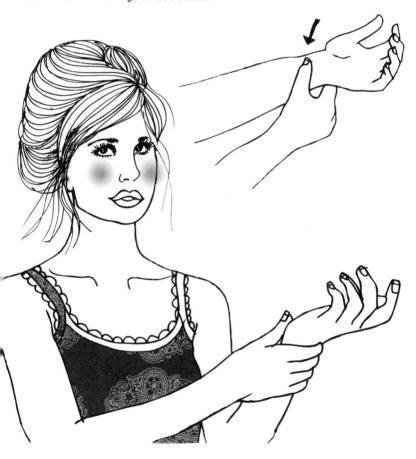

NECK STIFFNESS

TAKE A SIDEWAYS APPROACH

Inhale and then, as you exhale, slowly lower your right ear
towards your right shoulder (it won't reach so don't force it)
until there is a gentle stretch along the top of the left shoulder
and neck. Take several slow deep breaths. Inhale and raise your
head back up. Repeat on the other side.

FLEX YOUR NECK

For neck pain and stiffness that have been caused by muscle
tightening, gently move the neck to the outer ranges of its
movement while sitting in a comfortable chair. This will help
release muscle spasms and reduce the associated pain.

STRETCH AWAY STIFFNESS

For stiffness, inhale and then, as you exhale, slowly start to
lower your chin to your chest, giving yourself a long, gentle
stretch along the back of the neck. Take several slow, deep
breaths with the chin down and then lift your head back up again
on an inhale.

ROLL AWAY RIGIDITY

Lower one ear towards your shoulder, then roll your chin down
towards the chest, across the chest and up the other side. Inhale
and then, as you exhale, roll your chin down across the chest
and up the other side.

MASSAGE PROBLEMS AWAY

Applying warmth and gentle massage to sore and stiff necks can help reduce pain and increase healing blood flow.

SHRUG OFF NECK PROBLEMS

Inhale and raise your shoulders up to your ears, pulling them up as high as they'll go. Then let go with an 'ahhh' and drop your shoulders slowly back down. Repeat several times to ease muscle tension.

STAY IN THE SWIM

The best exercise to ease a stiff neck is swimming on your back. The water supports the head without straining the neck, allowing muscles to be used and stretched without discomfort.

FORM A SHOULDER CIRCLE

Raise your shoulders up, rotate them back and down, then forwards and up again. Repeat several times, then go in the opposite direction.

PAIN

SAY BYE-BYE TO RSI

An estimated one in 50 people suffer some form of RSI (Repetitive Strain Injury), which is caused by repetitive overuse of the soft tissue muscles of the neck, back, shoulders, arms and hands. Most of these injuries could be avoided altogether simply by taking short, regular breaks throughout the day.

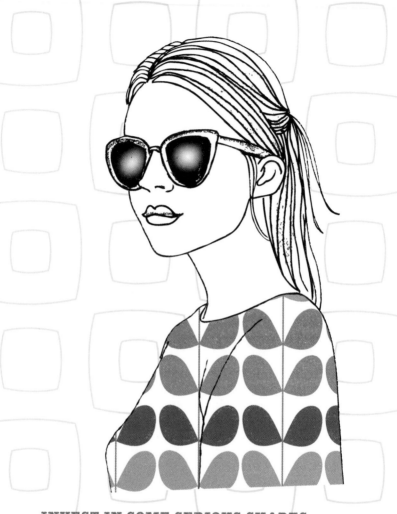

INVEST IN SOME SERIOUS SHADES

To prevent eye pain and potential damage, don't skimp on proper
eye protection – get a good pair of optical-grade, polarized
sunglasses that don't have the distortion associated with some
types of cheap lenses. Polarization is essential for cutting glare
and reducing eyestrain.

THINK YOURSELF SOFT

Focus on the part of your body that is feeling tense or is generating pain. What image comes to mind? Perhaps you see a rock or a tight knot. This represents receptive imagery. Try turning it into something soft, such as clay, or change the colour you perceive it to be, and feel your pain begin to dissolve away.

REACH OUT FOR HEALING HANDS

Massage decreases stress hormones, which can be a contributing factor to pain. It also seems to increase levels of endorphins, which are natural painkillers.

GO ALL-NATURAL

MSM (methyl-sulphonyl-methane) is an organic form of sulphur that has been shown to alleviate pain without producing side effects. It is found naturally in fruits, vegetables, meat, milk and seafood and seems to be particularly effective at easing muscle cramps.

DON'T SKIP MEALS IF YOU WANT TO SKIP PAIN

Skipping meals can result in increased pain, possibly because of fluctuations in blood sugar levels in the body brought on by long periods without nourishment. Always take a healthy snack along with you if you know you will be too busy to make time for a proper meal.

MAGNIFY MAGNESIUM

Soya beans, wholegrains, nuts, seeds, vegetables and fish all contain magnesium, which is an effective muscle relaxant shown to reduce tension pain. Lack of magnesium has been linked to depression, muscle soreness and general pain.

BLOW HOT AND COLD

Warmth can relieve pain by relaxing muscles. In contrast, cold relieves pain by reducing inflammation. Alternating between the two can help many types of muscle pain.

PEPPER YOURSELF WITH A CURE

Cayenne pepper contains a substance called capsaicin, which stimulates the brain to secrete endorphins, peptides that help block pain signals and reduce chronic pain, such as that from arthritis and bad backs. Sprinkle the cayenne pepper in hot water for a cure with a kick.

SOOTHE SKIN WITH CALENDULA

Calendula is an excellent herb for reducing the pain of most skin disorders, including nappy (diaper) rash, sunburns, bruises, and insect stings and bites. The herb has a calming, soothing effect on irritated skin by reducing inflammation and combating any associated infection, and there are topical skin ointments and creams available.

BE A PAIN-FREE WATER BABY

Even mild dehydration can trigger pain, so drinking lots of fluids is essential for pain-free living. The head is especially affected, but muscle pain, cramps and eyestrain can be caused by dehydration, too.

FIGHT INFLAMMATION WITH FOOD

Some types of food have natural anti-inflammatory properties that can reduce swelling and, therefore, alleviate pain. The best options for you to try are avocado, banana, berries, cabbage, cucumber, fig, mango and melon.

STEER CLEAR OF TRIGGERS

Some types of foods may actually increase the perception of pain, possibly because of their capacity for raising acid levels in the body. So, if you are suffering from persistent pain, cut down on alcohol, coffee, citrus fruits, onions, chocolate, sugar and salt.

STOMACH PROBLEMS

GO FOR A WALK

Exercise helps move gas through the digestive tract. That's why experts suggest that you take a short walk after eating instead of taking a nap. Mint tea can also aid digestion.

SETTLE THE STOMACH WITH MILK

Artichokes and milk products can help indigestion caused by too much stomach acid by lining the inside of the stomach after overeating or excessively rich food.

SWAP THE FRIES

French fries, red meat, sugar and refined grains in foods can increase the risk of colon cancer in women who eat them regularly. Replacing these foods with healthier alternatives like wholegrains, boiled or baked potatoes and low-sugar options could help cut your risk of colon cancer by half.

GO FOR PEPPER INSTEAD OF MILK TO CURE ULCER PAIN

Calcium in milk could make ulcer pain worse instead of better. To cure ulcers, steer clear of alcohol and spicy foods except capsaicin, a pepper derivative that seems to help ulcer pain.

RUB AWAY THE BLOAT

Try stroking gently from your right hip up towards your ribs,
across the bottom of your ribcage and down towards your left hip.
Repeat several times to encourage the movement of trapped wind.

TIRED ALL THE TIME

KEEP ZIPPING ALONG

Fatigue is one of the first symptoms of dehydration. Increase
your daily intake of water by drinking a glass with each meal
and sipping throughout the day.

TRASH THE CRASH DIET

Low-calorie consumption is a major cause of fatigue in women
today. Those who diet frequently may not have enough fuel to
sustain their body's optimal efficiency level, leading to tiredness
and fatigue.

DON'T COUNT ON CAFFEINE

Caffeine mimics the effects of stress hormones in the body. A
person who weighs 70kg (11st/154lb) and drinks more than six
caffeine drinks per day (for example, six cups of coffee or cola)
can develop caffeine 'poisoning', with symptoms of restlessness,
irritability, headache, insomnia and tiredness.

DO A SLEEP SURVEY

Lack of sleep or bad-quality sleep is a prime cause of tiredness.
Keep track of the hours you sleep and note irregularities. Make
sure your room is dark and quiet and don't carry stresses to bed
with you.

DON'T DISMISS DEPRESSION

One of the major symptoms of depression is extreme tiredness, so if you feel fatigued all the time you might want to consider depression as an underlying cause. Consult your doctor if you need advice.

CAN TIREDNESS WITH SARDINES

Tiredness can be a result of low iron, which also leads to cracked lips, cold hands and feet, poor memory, headaches, poor resistance to infection and pallor in the face and inner eyelids. Eat iron-rich sardines to boost energy.

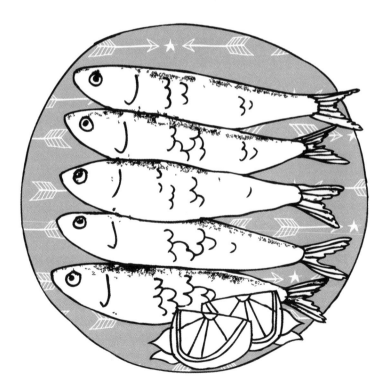

B WISE TO ENERGIZE

Adequate supplies of vitamins and minerals are essential for healthy metabolism. If these become in short supply for any reason, you will soon experience persistent tiredness. The B group of vitamins is especially important, as it's needed to produce energy.

ASK THE EXPERTS

If you feel tired all the time (known as TATT) for longer than two weeks, despite increasing exercise levels, eating a healthy diet and improving your quality of sleep, you must see your doctor. Tiredness is an early symptom of many illnesses, including thyroid problems and multiple sclerosis.

DON'T LET HORMONES WEAR YOU OUT

Low oestrogen levels can cause tiredness, especially when hormone levels drop in the week before your period or during the menopause, when tiredness can be overwhelming. Some studies have shown that regular carbohydrate snacks can help prevent this feeling.

STUB OUT THE CIGGY

Smoking affects everything to do with your body, increasing dehydration and stress levels and generating a whole range of metabolic problems. Heavy smokers often feel tired due to a lack of oxygen in their bloodstream.

LEAP INTO ACTION

Lack of exercise is one of the key causes of low energy and feelings of constant tiredness. Inactivity can also encourage weight gain and this in turn is likely to make you feel depressed.

MAKE A MENTAL NOTE

If you are worrying that you haven't completed some chore or important task, make a mental note that you are going to do it and when, which will help your brain stop worrying about it.

GET YOUR TIMING RIGHT

Organizing your life better can help you build in more opportunities for relaxation. Aim to balance all the aspects of your life, scheduling in time for your domestic chores and job as well as your social activities.

WATERWORKS

DON'T PEE TOO OFTEN

Going to the toilet too frequently can weaken your bladder by causing muscle fatigue, while women who crouch over the toilet are less likely to empty their bladders fully and are at risk of infection.

DON'T FORCE IT

If you feel the need to go to the toilet but once you get there you're as dry as a bone, you could have a urinary tract infection. Consult your doctor straight away in order to prevent the problem spreading to the bladder and kidneys and becoming even more serious.

GET THE ALL-CLEAR

Aim to drink enough water to make your urine pale yellow and clear. Dark yellow or cloudy urine is a sign that you aren't consuming enough fluid, so drink up.

JACK IN THE PACK

Smoking increases the risk of urinary tract conditions as well as raises blood pressure and stimulates coughing, which can add to problems with bladder control. It also increases the risk of bladder cancer, a risk that can stay with you for years after you have quit smoking.

STAY OFF STRONG STIMULANTS

Coffee, alcohol, spicy foods, citrus fruits and chocolate can all aggravate bladder problems, making urine more concentrated and so forcing the body to expend water in order to detoxify itself.

GET IT DOWN TO A TEA

Drinking tea made from raspberry leaves has been shown to reduce the pain and duration of urinary tract infections, and it is especially effective if taken regularly as problems begin.

SIT DOWN AFTER SEX

During sexual intercourse, bacteria may enter the urethra. By going to the toilet straight afterwards, you help wash out the invaders right away and avoid infections.

WIPE AWAY PROBLEMS

Keep infections at bay by cleaning the vaginal area with a front-to-back motion, which helps prevent the spread of bacteria from the anus.

HALT THE FLOW TO STAY STRONG BELOW

When you pee, practise stopping and starting the flow using your pelvic floor muscles to keep them tight and strong, Don't overdo it, though – three times a day is enough to help build muscle strength.

AVOID THE FIZZ

Fizzy mineral water can exacerbate some urinary tract conditions, so if you want to stay pain-free, have plenty of still, clear water to flush out the problems.

CHOOSE CRANBERRIES FOR CYSTITIS

Women have known this for years, but drinking cranberry juice regularly can help ease the symptoms of cystitis, possibly because it alters the acidity levels of the urine.

EAT TO CURE URINARY INFECTIONS

Health-inducing blueberries are rich in the bacteria-killing anthocyanosides, which will also see off the dreaded E. coli infections by preventing the infectious bacteria from clinging to the cells that line the urinary tract and bladder.

WOMEN'S HEALTH

MENOPAUSE

EAT YOUR GREENS

Postmenopausal women who have an excess of animal foods
in their diet are more likely to have low bone density, because
of the high acid levels in meat. Vegetables will counteract the
acidity of meaty dishes, so it's important to eat a balanced diet.

HERBAL REMEDY FOR HOT FLUSHES

The herbal supplement black cohosh has been found to alleviate
menopausal symptoms, such as hot flushes, sleep disturbance
and depressive moods, when taken daily.

STAY SOYA STRONG

Menopausal women who eat soya benefit from a noticeable
lessening of upsetting symptoms as well as a lower risk of bone
disease because of the bone-strengthening effects of the food.

COOL DOWN WITH VITAMINS

Many women claim to have experienced beneficial effects from
taking vitamin E for hot flushes and vitamin B2 for headaches.

MINIMIZE MOOD SWINGS

St John's Wort is effective in treating mood swings as well as
mild depression. Liquorice is thought to help hot flushes but it
can increase blood pressure so, as with all herbal preparations,
use it with caution.

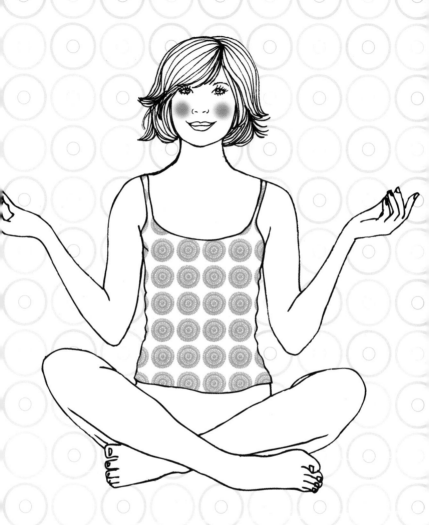

DON'T SWEAT IT WITH YOGA

Yoga and the Alexander Technique can reduce menopausal symptoms such as hot flushes and night sweats, while relaxation techniques, such as meditation and visualization, may assist by relieving mental and physical stress.

POP CORN TO POP DEPRESSION

A slight drop in the levels of the 'feel good' brain chemical serotonin could be one of the causes of depression during the menopause. A high-carbohydrate, low-fat snack, such as fat-free popcorn, may help restore serotonin levels in the brain, thereby improving your mood.

NATURAL HRT

Phytoestrogens are oestrogen-like compounds that are found in soya beans. They seem to bind to oestrogen receptors and act in a similar way to the female hormone in the body, reducing the incidence of hot flushes by up to 40%.

HAVE FUN WITH FUNGUS

Mushrooms, as well as onions, milk, garlic, eggs and seafood, contain selenium, which is an antioxidant mineral that can alleviate menopausal distress and allow you to smile through the flushes.

PERIODS

JOG AWAY PAIN

Taking regular exercise – for example, aerobics or jogging – can help reduce the symptoms of PMS (PMT). However, you should be exercising on a regular basis, not just when symptoms are present, if you want to enjoy the full health benefits.

EXPERIMENT WITH EPO

Some women find that taking evening primrose oil helps relieve breast discomfort. Long-term treatment (more than three months) may be required before any effect is noticed, however.

SMOOTHIE AWAY SYMPTOMS

Studies suggest that daily doses of magnesium and calcium taken during the time PMS (PMT) symptoms occur could have a cocktail of effects – helping reduce mood swings, muscle pains and fluid retention. Get both minerals at once in a soothing banana smoothie, made with either milk or yogurt.

SECURE A FISHY CURE

Fish fats help to relieve the symptoms of premenstrual disorders, including breast pain, PMT, bloating, depression and irritability. Choose oily fish such as mackerel, herring, sardines and salmon for the best effects.

IRON OUT PMT PROBLEMS

Heavy menstrual blood flow can deplete your body's iron stores, which can in turn cause further bleeding. Women who increase the iron in their diets are likely to suffer less heavy and painful periods. Sources include lean red meat, sardines, egg yolk, dried figs and dark green leafy vegetables like spinach.

PLANT THE SEEDS OF A CURE

Blackcurrant seeds, evening primrose seeds and borage seeds are all high in gamma linolenic acid (GLA), which helps regulate fluid retention and hormone release, helping minimize symptoms of PMS (PMT) and period problems.

SEND PMT CRAMPS BALMY

Lemonbalm is often used for menstrual problems as it has a calming and regulating effect in the menstrual cycle. It helps ease menstrual cramps and treats irregularities.

BEEF UP TO REDUCE CRAMPS

Supplementing the diet with zinc, found in high proportions in red meats like beef and lamb, has been found to reduce cramps, bloating and other PMS (PMT) symptoms.

STRENGTHEN WITH VITAMIN C

Taking vitamin C and bioflavonoids may strengthen uterine blood vessels and make them less susceptible to damage, so reducing the severity and length of bleeding during periods.

MANAGE WITH MARJORAM

Essential oil of marjoram has been shown to increase warmth and comfort if used to massage the abdomen during menstruation or in a burner to encourage pain-free sleep.

MASSAGE AWAY THE PAIN

Place your hands on your hips with the thumbs on the lower back at hip level, either side of the spine, and move the thumbs in small, light circular motions. Be gentle to avoid pain or discomfort.

PREGNANCY

DON'T EAT FOR TWO

Experts recommend that pregnant women need only an extra 300 calories a day to ensure the proper development of the foetus, and then only in the last three months. Energy requirements change little during pregnancy, so the effects of eating those extra calories are likely just to add weight to the mother.

SEAFOOD FOR A GOOD BIRTHWEIGHT BABY

Low consumption of seafood during the early stages of pregnancy may be a strong risk factor for low birthweight, because the omega-3 fatty acids they contain may help foetal development.

FOCUS ON FOLIC ACID

Folic acid lowers the chances that your baby will have spinal cord problems, so pregnant women should take a daily supplement before and during pregnancy until the twelfth week.

SWIM AWAY FROM PAIN

Swimming can help relieve many aches and pains and makes you feel weightless. This reduces pressure on the joints, hips and spine, which can become sore in the later months of pregnancy.

DON'T CURB CARBS

Mothers who eat more carbohydrates than fats while they're breast-feeding may have higher levels of a hormone known as leptin in their blood, which may later help them lose any weight that they gained during pregnancy. Carbohydrates are also essential for producing breastmilk.

TAKE VITAMINS TO VANQUISH TOXINS

Vitamins C and E fight off the symptoms of pre-eclampsia, a serious pregnancy-related condition that generates toxic compounds, raises blood pressure and endangers the life of mother and child. In studies, women taking a combined supplement had a 76% lower risk of developing the condition.

SNIFF AWAY LABOUR PAINS

Anxiety, pain, nausea and vomiting during labour can all be helped by using aromatherapy. The scents of ginger and citrus fruits are good for nausea, while bergamot, eucalyptus and pine are thought to lessen pain.

BRUSH UP ON TOOTHCARE

Take extra care of your general oral hygiene, especially your teeth and gums, during pregnancy as they may become more prone to plaque, cavities and disease at this time. Daily flossing and regular brushing after meals with a soft-to-medium brush is the answer.

STRETCH OUT TIRED BACKS

The leg lift crawl is excellent for an aching back. To do this, kneel on your hands and knees. Slowly bring your right knee towards your right elbow. Then slowly straighten your leg and lift it up and back, parallel to the floor. Avoid sudden jerks and keep your back straight, not arched. Repeat with each leg five to ten times.

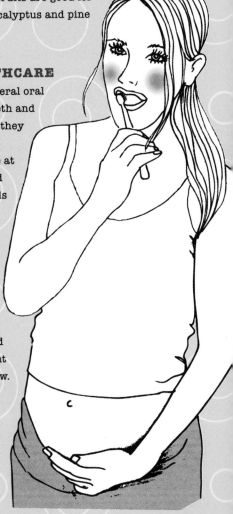

BE A WHITE WITCH

Witch hazel lotion and gel can reduce the pain and swelling of haemorrhoids. For further relief, try warm baths or use witch hazel compresses to ease severe swelling.

TILT YOUR PELVIS LIKE ELVIS

Taking exercise in the form of gentle pelvic tilts, using the muscles of your lower abdomen, will help relieve compression pain in your lower back, and it may even encourage the baby to assume a good birth position.

CAVE IN TO CRAVINGS

There is some evidence to suggest that food cravings may be your body's way of ensuring you get the vitamins and minerals you lack during pregnancy. So giving in to them might not be a bad thing – as long as you don't overeat.

TAKE IT EASY AT THE START

For the first three months, pregnant women should avoid overexertion and dehydration as this is a critical time for the baby and these conditions could harm development or trigger miscarriage.

BE A DAIRY LOVER

Regularly drinking more milk, or foods that substitute for milk, and eating more protein will help your baby's development in the womb by keeping your calcium at optimum level.

BODY CARE

CELLULITE

DRINK AWAY YOUR DIMPLES

Much cellulite is thought to be the result of an insufficient water intake. Drinking water plumps up the skin cells and smooths out subcutaneous dimpling. So if you want the smoothest possible skin, you should drink eight glasses a day.

DON'T CRASH AND BURN

Crash diets don't banish cellulite – in fact, they increase the risk because the body goes into starvation mode and holds on to fat, particularly in storage areas like the thighs and hips.

USE SUNFLOWERS TO SHRINK FAT

Fluid retention can result in the development of cellulite, as fluids become trapped in the fatty cells located under the skin. Linoleic acid, which is a substance found in sunflower and corn oils, may lessen fluid retention and so improve the appearance of cellulite.

GIVE TOXINS THE BRUSH OFF

Body brushing until the skin turns pink improves circulation to fatty areas, where blood flow is less efficient than in other areas of the body. This helps provide energy for healing and boosts the waste-removal process.

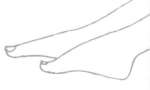

GIVE YOURSELF A HELPING HAND

Massaging your thighs and hips can help promote circulation
to fatty areas. Make sure the massage strokes always travel
upwards, towards the heart – in the direction of lymph clearance.

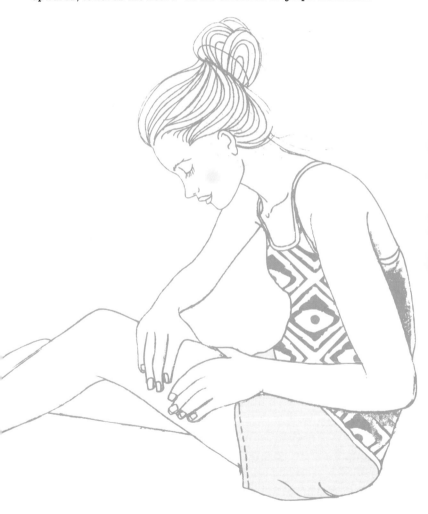

QUIT THE WEED TO SMOKE OUT DIMPLES

Smoking weakens the skin by causing constriction of the blood capillaries, worsening circulation and damaging the connective tissues, which in turn causes the dimpling effect of cellulite. Quit smoking to quash cellulite.

KEEP YOURSELF STIMULATED

Rubbing coffee grounds on areas affected by cellulite might be the supermodel's favourite trick, but it doesn't have to be coffee. The benefits are due to the skin stimulation, which boosts circulation and works toxins away from fatty areas.

GO GREEN TO BURN AWAY FAT

Studies have shown that drinking three cups of green tea a day can help reduce cellulite by boosting baseline metabolism and helping the body eliminate toxins. The caffeine it contains has a further stimulating effect.

WORK IT OUT

Exercise not only promotes overall health, but also works to improve muscle tone and circulation and frees up blocked tissue to remove the appearance of cellulite.

PILL A FAST ONE

Contraceptive pills raise oestrogen levels and can make fat cells enlarge and retain water, leading to cellulite. Diuretics, diet and sleeping pills can all make it worse.

GO LEAN FOR THINNER THIGHS

Saturated fats build cellulite and block arteries, and they can get trapped in the body's tissues, preventing waste and toxin elimination and encouraging fatty deposits.

HAIR & SCALP

DITCH THE ITCH
Ease an itchy, flaky scalp with a relaxing tea tree oil head massage to stimulate circulation in the scalp and help clear up dry and itchy skin.

RINSE, RINSE AND RINSE AGAIN
Many people confuse dried hair product with dandruff. For a healthy scalp, avoid heavy styling products and rinse thoroughly to avoid buildup.

SHINE UP WITH SWEET POTATO
Sweet potato, carrot and red pepper contain high levels of betacarotene, which the body needs to create vitamin A, essential to provide a protective layer to the outside of hair strands.

GET AHEAD WITH SOYA
Soya not only boosts hair health but has also been shown to make hair grow faster at the root and strengthen the shaft against damage.

MASSAGE FOR THICKER HAIR
Thinning hair and a lazy scalp can be stimulated by a weekly scalp massage. Use fingertips to rub small areas of the scalp at a time, remembering to include the hair-line, where dead skin cells can build up.

FIGHT THE FRIZZ

Coconut oil reduces frizziness and dryness in lacklustre hair, not only when used as a hair treatment but also when eaten. Coconut can be flaked or shredded and coconut milk can be used in cooking.

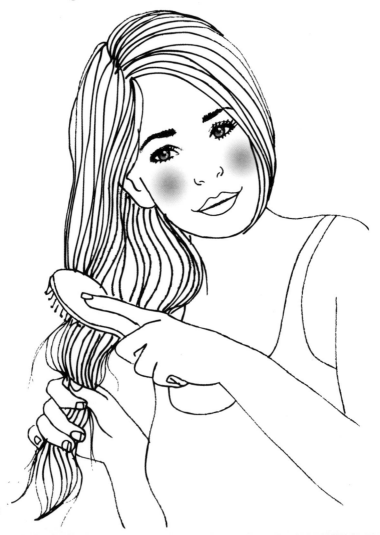

HANDS & FEET

BLISTERING HEALTH
Studies have shown that piercing a blister in the first three hours can help it heal. Use a sterile needle and lance as shallowly as possible in two places from opposite sides, treating to avoid infection.

ROLL AWAY STRESSFUL FEET
Feet can take a pounding during the day and a great way to relieve stress when you get home from work is to roll your feet over a cold soft-drink can to stimulate blood flow and reduce swelling.

SOFTEN OFTEN
The secret of dealing with hard skin on feet is to rub it away every day rather than at the odd irregular session. Use a pumice stone or file, softening the skin first by soaking in water with a teaspoon of bicarbonate of soda.

REACH FOR SOME LEMON AID
The citric acid in lemon juice works as a natural bleaching agent for discoloured nail tips. Dip a cotton bud (swab) in neat lemon juice and work it under the nail, then rinse after ten minutes for super-clean nails.

FOIL FLAKINESS WITH STARFLOWER OIL
Flaky nails can be sprung back into health by including starflower or evening primrose oil in the diet or as a supplement. Both contain the essential fatty acids (EFAs) necessary for the structure of cells.

IRON OUT FLAT NAILS

Too little iron in the diet can lead to thin, flat nails so increase your iron intake by eating foods such as lean red meat, dried fruit and nuts and green vegetables.

CHECK YOUR RIDGES

Ridges running across your nails could be a sign that stress is affecting your body in adverse ways. If your nails feel rippled, think about giving yourself time to relax.

BRUSH UP FOR CLEAN HANDS

Brushing your fingertips with toothpaste can remove nicotine or ink stains. Use a nailbrush to work the toothpaste into the skin for a few minutes, then rinse off.

GET PRIMROSE-STRONG NAILS

Evening primrose oil is essential for strong, hardy nails, and getting enough calcium, iron, zinc, protein and vitamins A, B and C is important as well.

CLOCK THOSE SOCKS!

Feet perspire more than any other area of the body, with each foot containing around 25,000 sweat glands and producing an eggcup of sweat every day. Wearing socks in natural or wicking materials helps them stay dry and healthy.

WATCH OUT FOR CLUBBING

Clubbing is when fingertips widen and become round, with nails curved around the fingertips. This serious condition is the result of an enlargement in connective tissue and can be a sign of an underlying lung disease. You must consult your doctor for advice.

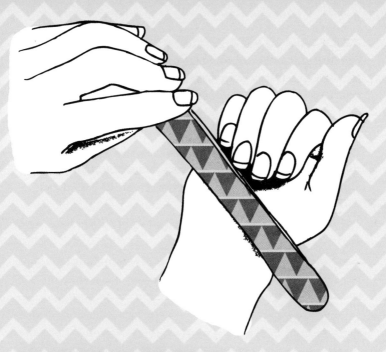

ALLOW NAILS TO BREATHE

A couple of days a month give your nails some time off polish
so they can breathe. Buffing during this time will give them a
natural shine and boost circulation.

WATCH OUT FOR BEAU'S LINES

Beau's lines are indentations that run across the nail and appear
when growth at the matrix is disturbed. This can happen after
illness or prolonged periods of stress.

GO FISHY TO CURE WHITE SPOTS

Eat foods rich in sulphur and silicon, such as broccoli, fish, royal
jelly, kelp and onions, which will help preserve nail colour and
keep cuticles pink and strong.

PUSH THE RIGHT BUTTONS

Nails and fingertips can suffer when in constant contact with keyboards for typing. Give them a rest by stretching out hands and shaking fingers to reduce tension.

KEEP IT TOGETHER

When the nail separates from the nail bed, this can be a sign that something is wrong, such as psoriasis, fungal infection, contact dermatitis or an adverse drug reaction. It can also be a sign of thyroid problems.

AVOID THE CUT

Never cut cuticles, because they will only grow back thicker if you snip them off. Instead, warm up hands in warm water or steam and gently push back cuticles with a cuticle stick.

DON'T DIG UP TROUBLE

Don't dig under nails to clean them, which damages the thin protective underlayer. Instead, use a soft nailbrush or an old toothbrush to get to hard-to-reach areas.

SKIN HEALTH

EAT FISH TO FIGHT FLAKY SKIN

Flaky, dry skin could signal that you are not getting enough essential fatty acids (EFAs), found in certain fish, seeds, nuts and oils. Healthy skin should contain about 15% fatty acids, so make sure you eat at least four portions of EFA-rich foods a week.

QUIT SMOKING TO KEEP SKIN SUPPLE

Smokers have saggier skin than non-smokers because of the damage done to their skin's elastin by the oxidative elements found in smoke, and because smoking impedes circulation.

ANTIOXIDANTS TO FIGHT AGEING

Antioxidants in vitamin A (sources include vegetables and fruit such as tomatoes, carrots, sweet potatoes, watermelons and apricots) combat free radicals that may lead to premature skin ageing and disease.

C IS FOR COLLAGEN

Vitamin C is essential for the growth of new collagen, which keeps the structure of your skin supple and firm and young-looking. Without it, skin will start to sag and look tired and old. So make sure you get enough in your diet and stop smoking, as it reduces vitamin C absorption.

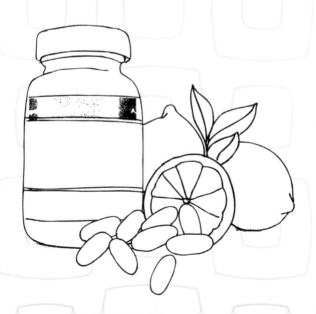

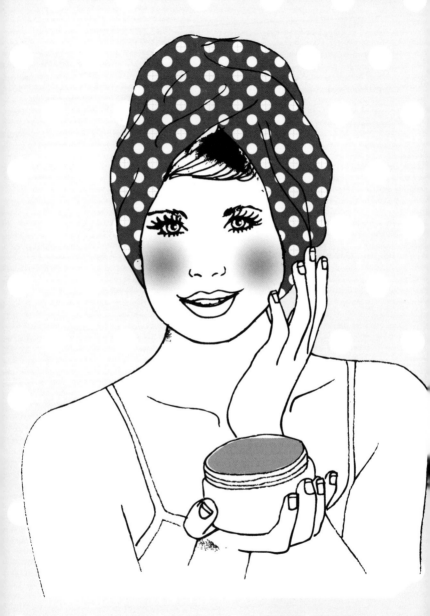

WITCH HUNT FOR HEALTHY SKIN

Witch hazel has anti-inflammatory properties that can help soothe and heal minor skin irritations, inflammation of the skin and mucous membranes, varicose veins and haemorrhoids when applied directly, and gum problems when diluted as a mouth rinse.

SEED THE DIFFERENCE

The omega-6 fats, which are derived exclusively from seeds and their oils, are essential for skin health, keeping it firm and moisturized. The best sources of omega-6 fats are hemp, pumpkin, sunflower, sesame, walnut and primrose oils, which can be included in the diet or as an element in beauty regimes.

TREAT PALE SKIN WITH IRON

Nearly 18% of women suffer from a lack of iron. If the skin appears pale and thin, this could be the problem. The richest sources are red meat, tuna and sardines, and the body also has the ability to convert lentils into iron.

ATTACK ACNE WITH PRIMROSE OIL

Take linseed (flaxseed) oil or evening primrose oil – which are both good sources of essential fatty acids (EFAs) – every day to rebalance the skin oils and to prevent the excess sebum production that can result in the development of acne.

E-LIMINATE DERMATITIS

Atopic dermatitis, a skin disorder characterized by redness, itching, eczema and thickening of the skin, can be soothed and even cured by a daily dose of the antioxidant vitamin E, found in avocado, seeds, nuts and supplements.

EAT AWAY SPOTS AND INFECTIONS

Zinc is essential for a healthy immune system and for fighting spots and skin blemishes. Found in red meat, oysters, peanuts and sunflower seeds, this mineral helps reduce the risk of skin infections, spots and boils.

TRY TEA TREE

Tea tree oil can help relieve acne and is also active against other skin problems, including fungal infections and cuts, bruises and bites. Manuka honey – made from tea tree sap – is also a powerful antiseptic with moisturizing qualities.

B GOOD TO YOUR SKIN

Vitamin B3 is an essential vitamin for healthy skin. Found in wholemeal bread and other wholegrain products, enriched breads and cereals, beef, chicken, nuts, peanut butter and salmon, it will help skin stay supple.

GO BLACK TO BASICS

Blackcurrant oil contains high levels of gamma linolenic acid (GLA), which promotes healthy, fast growth of skin, hair and nails. Use daily but expect to wait up to six weeks before you see visible results.

BE ROUGH TO BE SMOOTH

Exfoliation boosts blood flow to the skin, helps the skin renewal process and gets rid of dry skin cells that block and dull the complexion. Exfoliate with a gentle granular scrub once a week for the best results.

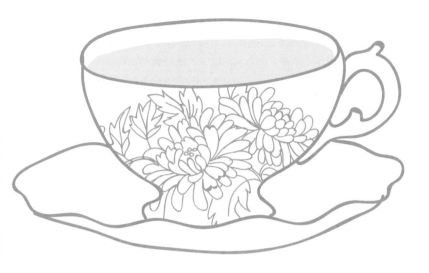

VOTE GREEN

Green tea, whether drunk or used as an ointment, reduces inflammatory responses and can help prevent skin problems.

GET A ROSY GLOW

Rosa mosqueta oil reduces scarring and blemishes, and can also help smooth wrinkles and plump up the skin's moisture levels to give it a natural, rosy glow.

GET A-GRADE SKIN

Foods that contain high levels of vitamin A, such as sweet potatoes, carrots, melons, red peppers, spinach, tomatoes, liver, fish, egg yolks, milk and other dairy products, boost general skin health and encourage regeneration of new skin.

LIQUIDIZE TO LICK SKIN INFECTION

Try this tip. Juice 4 carrots, 2 asparagus spears, half an iceberg lettuce and a handful of spinach leaves to protect your skin against infections and to maintain its suppleness. Drink this concoction three times a week.

DON'T YO-YO

Drastic weight fluctuations can stretch out the skin and cause it to sag. Avoid putting on or dropping too much weight for the best-looking skin long-term.

NOURISH SKIN WITH NUTS

Both walnuts and almonds are high in essential fatty acids (EFAs), which help replenish collagen, naturally moisturize the skin and promote youthful skin firmness. These nuts also contain anti-inflammatory properties that help keep skin smooth and pimple-free.

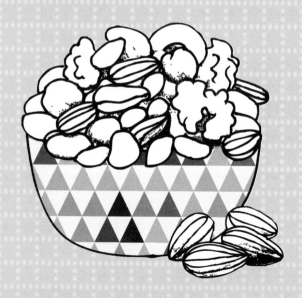

REPLICATE HIGH-TECH RETINOL

Retinol, which is the magic ingredient of expensive antiageing creams, is a form of vitamin A. Get your dose from the retinol in animal foods such as liver, oily fish, egg yolk, butter and cheese. The body converts retinol to vitamin A to build up collagen in deep skin layers.

BE A VIRGIN BEAUTY QUEEN

Extra-virgin olive oil contains strong antioxidants that combat the oxidizing effects of the sun on skin, reducing the signs of damage and ageing. Applying olive oil to the skin after sun exposure may help protect it.

GET YOUR BEAUTY SLEEP

Beauty sleep is not a myth. While you sleep, your skin regenerates and repairs itself. The peak time for moisture loss is 11pm to 4am. Older skin especially can suffer cell death if too much moisture evaporates, so make sure you go to bed well moisturized so the skin can heal itself.

SHIELD SKIN WITH SHEA

Shea butter contains incredibly high levels of vitamin E, which prevents oxidative damage to skin when applied regularly.

LOOK AFTER THIN SKIN

The skin on your face is the thinnest on the body, and the older the skin, the thinner and drier it can be. It will therefore need more protection and moisture, especially in the harsh winter months.

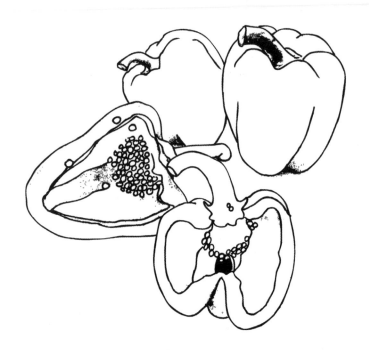

HEAL YOUR SKIN WITH PEPPERS

Both red and dark orange peppers are loaded with the antioxidant vitamins A and E and bioflavonoids, which help skin to heal from within.

OXYGENATE WITH GREEN LEAFYS

Like other green leafy vegetables, kale is rich in the antioxidant lutein and contains iron, which transports oxygen to your skin. It also contains vitamin A, which helps prevent premature wrinkling.

OIL UP WRINKLES WITH SALMON

Along with other coldwater fish like mackerel and tuna, salmon are rich in omega-3 fatty acids, which prevent inflammation and lubricate your skin.

SUN SAFETY

BEWARE OF AROMATHERAPY OILS

Some types of oils, including citrus oils like orange, lemon and bergamot, react with ultraviolet light from the sun and can cause skin to burn more easily, so beware of using them during summer months.

VITAL VITAMIN PROTECTION

Vitamins C and E may help protect the skin against sunburn and could possibly reduce the risk of skin cancer by neutralizing damaging free radicals that are produced by ultraviolet radiation coming from sunlight.

OPT FOR TOTAL COVER

When you're applying sunscreen, always remember not to miss hands, neck, ears and lips, which are common sites for skin cancer because of their propensity to burn.

KEEP YOUNG AND BEAUTIFUL

After smoking, sun exposure is the greatest wrinkle-creator for skin. Stay out of the sun or use moisturizing sunscreens with a high SPF factor to maximize your skin's chances of staying healthy and youthful.

TEETH

BE A SOFT TOUCH

Lots of gum problems are caused by brushing too vigorously, which can cause gums to retreat. Electric toothbrushes can tackle this by preventing hard pressing. If you're using a normal toothbrush, remember that bristles should bend only slightly against the tooth surface.

FLOSS AWAY DECAY

If you don't floss, you will leave an incredible 35% of the surface of your teeth completely untouched and uncleaned. So for really clean teeth, use thick tape and floss every night.

FILTER IN FLUORIDE

Fluoride is essential for healthy teeth, but some mineral waters contain low levels. Tap water is fortified, so make sure some of your water is filtered rather than bottled.

BE YOUR DENTIST'S FRIEND

Dentists recommend seeing a hygienist every three to six months as well as regular brushing. Make visits more often if you're diabetic, as you are more susceptible to gum disease.

GIVE YOUR MOUTH A RAW DEAL

Eating raw foods increases salivation and is good for tooth health. Choose neutral carrots and celery for the best results. Citrus fruits, because they contain so much citric acid, should be accompanied by a glass of water to wash away excess acids, which could attack your teeth.

DON'T RUSH TO BRUSH

It is best to leave about half an hour between eating and brushing your teeth to allow the mouth to build up its normal levels of saliva and bacteria again, as these act as a protective barrier over the tooth and gum surface.

A BRIGHT WHITE SMILE

For brighter teeth and to remove stains and plaque, wash your mouth out or brush with baking soda.

CHECK OUT THE CHEESEBOARD

Finishing off a meal with a piece of cheese can help protect your mouth against tooth decay, and even cooked cheese used as an ingredient in meals can help keep your teeth strong and healthy. At the end of a meal, the cheese protects dental enamel by lowering levels of mouth acidity.

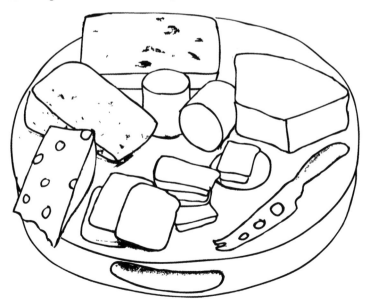

MIND OVER MATTER

BRAINPOWER

EAT A BRAINY BREAKFAST
The best food to boost your brainpower at breakfast is high-fibre, carbohydrate-rich food that releases energy slowly, such as wholegrain breads and cereals, porridge or fresh fruit, plus some protein from milk, bacon, eggs or peanut butter.

BE A DOUBLE-SIDER
Try using your other hand (your left hand if you're right-handed or your right if you're left-handed) for activities such as writing, eating and sports. Experts say that this will stimulate parts of your brain that routine habits cannot reach.

BANANAS ON THE BRAIN
The glucose released into the bloodstream from carbohydrates is the brain's favourite food, and the slower and steadier it's released, the better. Bananas, apples, porridge and stoneground bread are all good snacks.

DO SOME OLIVE GOOD THINKING
Both memory and concentration are better in people whose diets include high levels of monounsaturated fats, such as those that are to be found in olive and flaxseed oils. This is because of the beneficial effect these healthy fats have on the structure of brain-cell membranes.

WHIZZ UP SOME QUICK-FIX IQ FOOD

If you're feeling sluggish, whizz up a quick-fix brain boost, like a thought-boosting fruit smoothie with oats or apple purée and honey, which will keep your brain firing faster for longer.

BREATHE DEEP TO CLEAR YOUR HEAD

The brain is the body's second largest organ and uses 20% of the total oxygen pumping around your body. Make sure you feed it well with daily deep breathing exercises to boost oxygen circulation.

GET CREATIVE WITH CREATINE

Studies have shown that the dietary supplement creatine, used for building body muscle, could increase brainpower by maintaining a high energy flow to the brain.

IRON OUT MEMORY PROBLEMS

A deficiency of iron in the body will impair learning and memory skills along with cell growth in the rest of the body. To counter this, stock up on leafy green vegetables, figs, raisins, peas and meat, which contain high levels of the mineral.

BE A PILLOW LOVER

Sleep allows your brain to regenerate, keeping you clear-headed and bright throughout the following day. Experts think that between seven and eight hours a night is best for optimal brainpower.

GET FIT TO THINK

Approximately 750ml (1¼ pints) of blood pumps through your brain every minute of the day and night, and you can boost your potential brainpower simply by increasing the efficiency of your heart by introducing a 30-minute exercise programme into your routine three times a week.

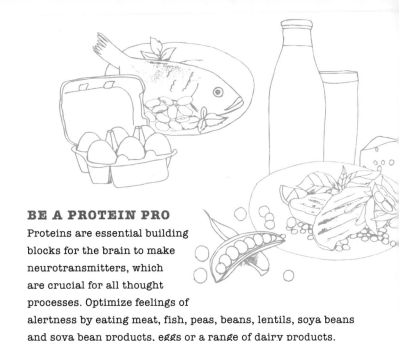

BE A PROTEIN PRO

Proteins are essential building blocks for the brain to make neurotransmitters, which are crucial for all thought processes. Optimize feelings of alertness by eating meat, fish, peas, beans, lentils, soya beans and soya bean products, eggs or a range of dairy products.

BE BERRY CLEVER

A cup of blueberries a day could improve short-term memory by protecting against age-related mental decline.

BREAKFAST LIKE A KING

People who have a proper meal at breakfast tend to have better reaction times, problem-solving abilities and a more acute memory than people who skip, skimp on or rush through their first meal of the day. So make time to breakfast royally.

FISH FOR MEMORIES

Shellfish contain zinc, which boosts short-term memory and recall as well as enhances verbal and visual memory. Zinc is also found in beans, dark turkey meat and peas.

BE AN ALL-DAY GRAZER

The brain needs nourishment 24 hours a day as it cannot store significant reserves of energy to keep it working. Missing a meal is detrimental to your thought processes, so aim to eat little and often to keep the brain's energy levels topped up.

GIVE YOUR BRAIN A WORKOUT

Each day, pick an object and study it for several minutes, then shut your eyes and recreate the image. Remember as much as you can, then open your eyes and see how much you missed. Repeat with different objects daily to boost concentration.

SHUN FAT TO STAY SHARP

High intakes of saturated fat could put people at greater risk of cognitive impairment. The healthiest diets for sharp brains are those containing oily fish like salmon and mackerel, which not only prevent degeneration of mental faculties but actually boost brainpower too.

SANDWICH SOME REST TIME

Carbohydrate foods, including starchy vegetables, pasta, potato, cereals and bread, stimulate the release of the relaxation chemical serotonin in the brain, which enables your brain to wind down after a long day.

GO MENTAL WITH MINERALS

Both sodium and potassium are vital ingredients when it comes to the optimal functioning of the brain, enhancing connections between neurons. Bananas are a tasty snack and high in potassium, while sodium is readily found in salt, meat and many other foods.

GET A MEATY REMINDER

Foods that are rich in protein, such as meat, fish, cheese, soya products and nuts, help the brain create dopamine, which is an essential chemical for quick thinking. Eating 75g–125g (3oz–4oz) of protein should help make you more alert and energized.

GET A BEANY BRAIN

Beans, peas, apples and pears contain high levels of boron, which helps enhance alertness and memory power.

NIBBLE NUTS FOR MEMORY

Nuts – particularly walnuts and brazil nuts – are full of the memory-boosting substance magnesium, which can improve brain function and alertness.

GO SLOW FOR QUICK THINKING

Low-density carbohydrate vegetables such as broccoli, spinach and pak choi, fresh herbs and low-glycaemic fruits like berries and melons release sugars slowly and help the brain work hard all day.

MAKE MINE AN ESPRESSO

Caffeine may improve memory by making existing brain cells swell and new ones grow, but too much can cause attention problems, so stick to espresso, which has less caffeine per serving than other coffees.

CHOOSE CHEESE FOR A CHAMPION BRAIN

Cheese can help to increase levels of the neurotransmitter acetylcholine in the brain, which assists general functioning. Other foods you can eat that do the same job include liver, fish, milk, broccoli, cabbage and cauliflower.

EAT SMALL FOR BIG SUCCESS

After a big meal, most of the body's oxygen is taken up by the intestines as they deal with the process of digestion, which means the brain gets less. This is why you often feel sleepy after a blow-out business lunch. If you want to stay alert to clinch that deal, eat light at lunch.

ADDRESS STRESS TO GET AHEAD

Stress hormones like cortisol destroy brain cells, which means the more stressed you are, the fuzzier your head will be. Allowing yourself to relax will help you concentrate.

BE YOUR OWN HERO

If you feel your confidence slipping at a business meeting or in a social situation, just think of someone you respect and admire and spend a few minutes acting like them. Eventually it will become second nature and their self-assurance will become part of your own.

BECOME SOYA CLEVER

Soya and soya products contain high levels of lecithin, which is essential for forming the structures of the brain, so make sure you include them in your diet.

DON'T SAY NO

Your brain does not understand negatives, so telling yourself not to think about something simply will not work. Instead, distract yourself by concentrating fully on something else and you will find that the worrying thought disappears.

RISE TO THE CHALLENGE

Challenging normal routines occasionally, like enrolling on a new course or feeling your way around your bedroom with your eyes shut, improves reaction times by forcing the brain to work harder.

GIVE YOURSELF A VEGETARIAN BRAIN BOOST

Vegetarians needing a brain boost could get instant benefits by upping the levels of protein (from nuts and soya) in their food or by taking a protein supplement, both of which will help stimulate the flow of blood to the brain.

REMEMBER TO ADD GARLIC

Garlic has been shown to improve spatial memory and to help protect against age-related memory loss. Use it in sauces, Italian-style meals and stir fries. confidence

STAND UP TO FEEL OUTSTANDING

Standing up straight encourages you to breathe more deeply, which will in turn reduce anxiety levels and help you feel more confident.

CALM DOWN WITH VALERIAN

The herb valerian has been shown to help more than two-thirds of people with anxiety. Make tea infusions from roots or take supplements when you feel low.

ACCENTUATE THE POSITIVE

The next time you catch yourself having a negative thought, however small, make an effort to turn it into a positive one. Negative thinking is a bad habit that needs to be broken, and conquering the small negatives is the best way to do it.

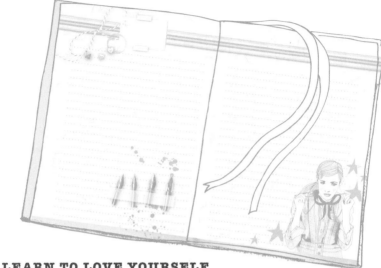

LEARN TO LOVE YOURSELF

Make a list of at least five to ten things you like about yourself
and carry the list around with you so you can refer to it when
your self-image is low.

NEGATE NERVES WITH A SNACK

If you feel sick with nerves, it could be because your stomach
is empty. Confidence levels drop when we're in need of food, so
have a healthy snack even if you think you're not hungry.

SALUTE THE SUN

Sunlight boosts the body's natural levels of mood-boosting
serotonin, so if you're feeling low on confidence a breath of fresh
air could be just what you need.

CURTAIL THE CAFFEINE

Caffeine increases heart rate, which can increase nervousness
and anxiety. If you want to feel cool, calm and collected, opt for
water or herbal tea instead.

DEPRESSION

MEDITATE YOUR MOOD AWAY

Meditation can help alleviate depression by relaxing the body
and reducing anxiety levels, especially if performed with
breathing exercises. Aim for at least ten minutes a day for
maximum benefits.

LOOK ON THE SUNNY SIDE

Giving yourself a good dose of sunlight is imperative to help fight
off the effects of depression, especially in the winter months,
when natural daylight is in short supply. Place your desk
beside a window and try to spend at least ten minutes outside
at midday. If the sun is strong, however, make sure you protect
your skin from the damaging effects of UV radiation.

BREATHE BERGAMOT TO FEEL BRIGHTER

For an instant mood boost, slip a few drops of bergamot essential
oil into your bath or an essential oil burner. Be careful if it's
sunny, however, as bergamot can increase sensitivity to sunlight.

HAPPINESS

WORK OUT THOSE WORRIES

Not only is it excellent for your body, exercise is also good for
your mind, stimulating the release of endorphins, which are the
natural hormones for producing a feeling of happiness.

FEED ON FEEL-GOOD FRUIT

Fruits containing high levels of vitamin C, like oranges, blackcurrants and kiwi fruit, can improve mood by encouraging your body to produce feel-good endorphins.

MOTIVATION

DO IT IN INTERVALS

If you struggle mentally to keep going during your workout, you might want to switch to interval training instead. Using this method, your brain may respond better to short bursts of activity, so enabling you to work harder for longer.

GIVE YOURSELF GOALS

Setting yourself achievable goals to aim for throughout the day will help your body enter a natural cycle of effort and reward. Remember to reward yourself by allowing yourself a few minutes off every time you achieve something, rather than rushing on to the next task.

NEGATIVE THOUGHTS

MAKE A THOUGHT CHAIN

Carry around a pocketful of paperclips and every time you have a negative thought about yourself, simply hook another paperclip onto the chain. At the end of the day, you might well be amazed to discover just how negative you are. Once you've identified your negative triggers, work at transforming them into positive ones.

LOCK AWAY NEGATIVITY

Start keeping a negative notebook in which to lock away destructive thoughts. Every time you think negatively, write the thought down and leave it there so the notebook gets filled up, instead of your brain.

A THOUGHT FOR THE DAY

Start every day with a positive thought about yourself. It could be something you like or enjoy doing, or something you feel – just as long as it's positive.

RELAXATION

TAKE THREE DEEP BREATHS

Put one hand on your chest and the other on your stomach. Take a deep breath in and feel the hand on your stomach move but the hand on your chest remain still. Exhale and then take a deep breath in and hold it for a count of three. Exhale through your mouth and count to five before taking the next deep breath.

ALL-OVER MUSCLE RELAXATION

Starting with your toes, tighten the muscles until they start to ache. Then completely relax, letting the toes go limp. Repeat this with all the major muscle groups – legs, arms, shoulders, neck – then the hands. Learn the difference between tense and relaxed, and when you feel tense, do a body check to see which muscles need relaxing.

TAKE TIME TO STAY CALM

Daily meditation has been shown to reduce stress levels and boost your body's immunity, so spend a couple of minutes meditating every morning, concentrating on breathing and emptying your mind of extraneous thoughts.

SEASONAL AFFECTIVE DISORDER

D FOR DEPRESSION

In a trial, SAD sufferers who took 400 IU (international units) of vitamin D a day during the winter felt more enthusiastic, inspired and alert, probably because the vitamin raises levels of the mood-lifting brain chemical serotonin.

HERBAL HIGH

The mood-boosting effects of the herb St John's Wort were marked in almost half of those who took it in one study. It can have side effects, so check with your doctor before taking it.

STRESS

DON'T STRESS WITH ESPRESSOS

Beware of reaching for a cup of coffee in an attempt to reduce feelings of stress. Coffee raises adrenaline levels by more than a third to make you feel more stressed, especially if you drink it alone. Instead, opt for herbal tea or a glass of water to soothe your nerves.

FLEX YOUR FACE

Studies have shown that many women react to tension by clenching the jaw, which only makes stress worse. If you find yourself with a clenched jaw, stretch your facial muscles by opening your mouth and eyes in a look of surprise. Hold this expression for a few seconds before relaxing.

LIFESTYLE

AGEING

BE A HONEY IF YOU WANT TO STAY SHARP

Too much sugar in the diet has been found to leave damaging beta amyloid deposits in the brain, which can contribute to brain degeneration and Alzheimer's disease. Swap sugar for healthier alternatives like honey or maple syrup.

POWER UP YOUR MEMORY

Gingko biloba, a tree extract that has been used by the Chinese for about 2,800 years, improves mental function by soaking up harmful free radicals and improving neurotransmission within the brain, promoting good blood circulation and enhancing memory.

BAD HABITS

UNEARTH HIDDEN DIET HORRORS

Write down everything you eat for three days. Do you add a lot of butter, sauces or salad dressings? Rather than eliminating these foods, cut back your portions.

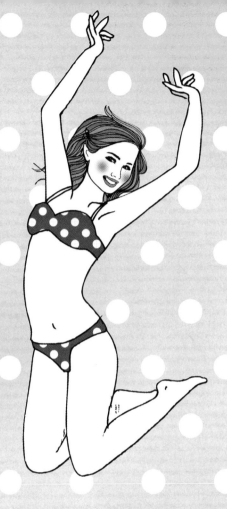

JUMP FOR BETTER JOINTS

Get into the high-impact habit. Studies have shown that to keep muscles and bones strong, resistance training that involves impact, such as running, walking, skipping rope and weight training, can be more beneficial than smooth, slow movements like swimming and cycling.

CLIMATE CHANGE

TURN OFF WHEN YOU TURN IN

Sleep quality and quantity are both better when the bedroom temperature is on the low side, so turning off the central heating or turning down the thermostat on winter nights could help you get a better night's sleep.

ESCAPE GERMS WITH ECHINACEA

Sudden, abrupt changes in the ambient temperature can take a toll on the body's energy levels, making it more prone to succumb to infections. If you're faced with hotter or colder climates, take echinacea, which has been shown to strengthen the immune system.

HANGOVERS

THINK QUALITY NOT QUANTITY

Cheaper brands of drinks often contain more toxins and are therefore harder for the liver to cope with, causing worse hangovers. Go for quality rather than quantity – the expense might motivate you to limit your drinking, too.

DETOX WITH A BEET DRINK

For a detoxifying antidote to all that partying, try beetroot juice mixed with the juices of carrot, apple, celery and ginger. The celery contains various antioxidant compounds that will help neutralize the effects of cigarette smoke, while the ginger will help relieve any nausea, stomachache or diarrhoea.

HAVE HONEY TO BURN OFF ALCOHOL

Before or while you're drinking, have a large glass of grapefruit juice, and eat some honey. The grapefruit is a liver tonic, and the honey helps your body burn off alcohol in your system.

BOOST YOUR B INTAKE FOR BETTER MORNINGS

Take a combination of B-complex vitamins, vitamin C and zinc before a night of drinking, and then again in the morning, to help your system replace what you have lost with your overindulgence. Research shows that your system turns to B vitamins when it is under stress, and alcohol depletes levels further.

DON'T SOBER UP WITH A COFFEE

Drinking caffeine, which is in its highest concentrations in filter coffee, is a diuretic and will rob your body of even more water and nutrients. Try water or a sports drink instead, to replace electrolytes and give you an energy boost.

SPICE UP YOUR LIFE

Ginger is one of the most effective natural remedies for nausea and indigestion, stimulating metabolism to encourage the elimination of toxins.

FEEL FINE AND DANDELION

The herb dandelion is a traditional liver tonic that has been shown to reduce the severity and duration of headaches.

PRESS YOUR LUCK

Try the ancient Chinese art of acupressure to relieve morning nausea. With your thumb, apply continuous pressure to the soft area between your thumb and index finger on either hand for several minutes.

MILK A CURE

Milk thistle is renowned for its ability to support and stimulate the working of the liver, which is the organ primarily responsible for detoxifying alcohol within the body. Take a dose of milk thistle before you go out and one when you get back for the best results.

BECOME AN ICE MAIDEN

Soothe a throbbing hangover headache the natural way with an ice pack. Soak cottonwool pads in cold camomile tea and then place them on your eyelids to reduce the swelling.

LIVE LONG & HEALTHY

THE PEEL-GOOD FACTOR

Adding more potassium to the diet can lower blood pressure, while a diet deprived of potassium can actually raise blood pressure. Eating one banana per day provides the extra 400mg of potassium needed to slash the odds of suffering a fatal stroke by 40%.

GIVE YOURSELF A RAW DEAL

According to studies, if you don't consume fruit daily, your risk of stomach cancer doubles or even triples, and raw is best. Munch on raw fruit and vegetables.

WEAR A COPPER

Copper is an essential supplement for reducing age-related disintegration of body tissues and it is an a nonallergenic material. Many people, particularly arthritis sufferers, wear copper bracelets for the absorption of the mineral into the skin.

HAVE A HEARTY DOSE OF ONION

Consuming half an onion a day, or the equivalent in juice, raises HDL (good) cholesterol by an average of 30% in most people with heart disease or cholesterol problems, extending life expectancy and boosting health.

LOVE

DON'T BE A PRUNE PRUDE

Not only are prunes top of the healthy, cancer-beater charts, they also have aphrodisiac properties. Eros, the Greek god of love, is said to have dipped his arrow in prune juice. You, however, can just eat them instead!

GET IN THE MED FOR LOVE

In the Mediterranean, pistachios and pine nuts are considered aphrodisiacs and certain spices, like cinnamon and nutmeg, are said to arouse both men and women.

SEX

ZINC INTO THE MOOD

A natural aphrodisiac and fertility booster, zinc is found in pumpkin and sesame seeds, cheese, chicken and turkey, wholegrains, pine nuts, brown rice, fish and seafood. Not forgetting (surprise, surprise) oysters!

TAKE TO THE FLOOR

Make your orgasms more powerful and work your pelvic floor muscles at the same time by contracting and relaxing them.

TAKE IODINE FOR LOW SEX DRIVE

In some people, low sex drive could be due to an underactive thyroid gland, so if you seldom feel in the mood, visit your doctor to have your thyroid checked; increased iodine could be the answer.

THYME FOR BED

Chromium, found in thyme, and also wholegrains, meat, cheese and brewer's yeast, is thought to increase sperm count in men and sex drive in both sexes.

TRAVEL

MOVE TO PREVENT MOTION SICKNESS

On a ship or plane, move to the centre where it tends to be more stable. On a ship, go to the top deck and look out at the water to put your eyes and inner ear in sync.

DRINK WATER, NOT ALCOHOL

Jetlag effects are generally made worse by dehydration, caffeine and alcohol, which put stress on the body and increase fatigue.

TREAT TRAVEL SICKNESS WITH GINGER

Ginger is a traditional herbal remedy and is available in pills, chewable ginger root and as sweets. Side effects seem to be minimal but it's always wise to check with your doctor since it has been shown to have some blood-thinning effects.

TREATS

BEAT YOUR TROUBLES WITH BUBBLES

Whenever time permits, indulge in a 30-minute 'home spa' session in your own bathroom. Soak your troubles away in your favourite bubble bath; lie back, close your eyes and let pleasant thoughts flood in.

SURROUND YOURSELF WITH FLOWERS

Research studies have shown that flowers provide an emotional lift. You don't need to spend a fortune to spread flowers throughout your house – buy one bouquet and split it up, putting a flower or two in several different vases.

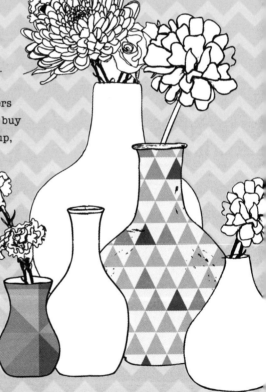

INDEX